LIGHT

— YOUR —

FIRE

IGNITE YOUR BURNING DESIRE
FOR A HEALTHIER YOU

A Simple Guide Toward
Longevity with Vitality

DR. JOSEPH K. JONES

Legal Disclaimer

Consult with your health care provider before making any changes to your diet or exercise regimen. Individual responses to diet and exercise protocols can vary. The information provided in this book is general in nature and may not be suitable for everyone. All information provided in the book is based on current scientific research and the best practices available. However, this book does not guarantee weight loss or other health outcomes. Results may vary depending on individual factors. Dr. Jones is not responsible for any losses, damage, or injuries that may result from the use of the information provided in this book.

ISBN:
Softcover: 978-1-956914-99-3
eBook: 978-1-961781-33-7

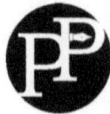

Dedicated to Mom

My mother, Helen T. Jones, passed away at 75 years young from COPD, a lifestyle-related disease. Her death, like the death of someone we've all loved and lost, came prematurely, before her eighth decade of life.

In her most recent inspirational book, *Shine Through Your Story*, Michelle Prince, a mentor of mine, talks of igniting our inner light to illuminate the world. This little lady, Helen, possessed an inner light that continues to shine even today, 11 years after her passing. Her light lit my passion to search for answers to the causes, solutions, and prevention of such early demises. Her light led me to fight misinformation and disinformation and inspire others to live with vitality and longevity. Her light led me to deliver this message: If we take care of our bodies and minds, a long life is more than possible.

Your life is your story. Don't let it be silenced in its second act. Live fully, until your entire story has been told—not just for you, but for all your loved ones who surround you. Let your life become your masterpiece.

Patient Testimonials:

I've had the privilege of having Dr. Jones as both my chiropractor and nutritionist for almost 10 years now. He has helped me correct a range of issues including lower back pain and reflux problems, and he's even helped me avoid various prescription medications. My back and reflux problems are completely gone! Dr. J. has educated me in what I need to do to stay healthy and feel good. His knowledge of health is amazing, and I feel truly blessed to know him!

–Anita Baroody

I have been a patient of Dr. Jones's for 18 years. He has been my first stop for all things related to my health. I am BEYOND thrilled that Dr. Jones has written a book that captures his vast knowledge and in-depth understanding of the human body. He possesses such wisdom pertaining to our bodily systems and how they relate to and respond to one another. It is quite literally mind-blowing. When you couple that with his understanding of how proper nutrition plays such an essential role in the vitality of these systems, you've got a goldmine! To now be able to hold this information in our own hands is very exciting.

–Karen Littlefield

The knowledge that Dr. Jones has on everything concerning nutrition and natural healing is astounding. I wish I had met the man years ago! I can truly say that I am becoming a better person day by day because of his instruction.

–Margaret Anderton

About four years ago, I started my journey of taking physical care of myself and, most importantly, changing my mindset about what I eat and how I move. The questions that Dr. Joseph Jones asks us to consider in the introduction to his book are ones I was initially afraid to answer. I was tired as soon as I woke up in the morning, and I especially hated looking in the mirror. It is scary to make changes in your life—and, yes, there are going to be good days and bad. But once you take that first step, you are well on your way. Dr. Jones gives a detailed plan on what you can do to make changes in the way you eat, and he discusses giving yourself grace if you do eat that piece of French bread. Although I have not met Dr. Jones, he gave me space to be okay, encouragement to make each day count, and the ability to make the best choices for myself. Thank you!

–Terese Ghilarducci

My health issues have been ongoing for about 15 years now. Through trial and error, and while dealing with allergies for my son and myself, I've learned to try certain things, see how my body reacts, and then proceed accordingly. My issues began with weakness in my leg; however, testing ruled out all endocrine-related disorders and showed my sugar level to be borderline high. A year later, I had a large tumor removed from my right ovary. My leg weakness subsided at first but then returned a year later along with hot flashes, irregular cycles, and a recurring cyst. Not long after, I was diagnosed with hidradenitis suppurativa. I have seen every type of doctor for all my symptoms, and while some of them would provide temporary relief, no one could offer a long-term solution.

I started seeing Dr. Jones a year ago, and since committing myself to his supplement protocol my breakouts are rare (depending on my eating habits). This result did not happen overnight. Learning to avoid triggering foods and trusting his supplement schedule have helped me achieve these goals.

–**Tabitha Fowler**

CONTENTS

ACKNOWLEDGMENTS

No book is written without the help of many. I would like to say a heartfelt thank you to a host of supportive people.

Leading acknowledgments must be given to Kimberly Kelsoe Hawkins. Thank you for sharing your "it!" I'm not certain if it was by mere fate or the grace of God that our paths crossed, but I am quite certain that this book would never have made it between its covers without your guidance and friendship. I am forever grateful for your awesomeness, your "it!"

To Stephanie Pitts—my right arm. Thank you for dissecting all my chicken scratch and making sense of what I was trying to say. I learned a valuable lesson early on in my life from observing my mom: "When you want to get something done, find the right women."

To Hanna E. Jones, my "Betcha-by-golly wow." A more beautiful site I've yet to see. To quote our daughters Bella and Audriana, you are the "best mommy ever."

To my brothers Dale and Tod, thanks for keeping it close for over half a century.

Thank you to Joseph Campanelli, my college roommate. You took me for my first chiropractic treatment and changed my life. Because of you, I changed my major to chiropractic and found my calling in life.

To Steven Oropeza, D.C. You have been a great mentor and inspiration throughout the years. Thank you.

To Bill DeCarlis, Tom Toulious, Paul Genet, and Sigmund Ringoen—know you are my Mount Rushmore.

Thank you to all my colleagues at Rocky Ridge Chiropractic throughout the last 30 years for your friendship, professional insights, and support.

To the many chiropractic patients throughout the years who found their calling as chiropractic physicians: May your hands continue to deliver health to all they touch.

Thank you to all my patients, friends, and colleagues who have inspired me and requested—and in some cases demanded—that I write this book.

Thank you to Standard Process for their dietary supplements, overall exceptional product line, and the vast knowledge they have shared with me throughout the years.

Thank you to Christopher Manning in appreciation of his time in reviewing the manuscript and his positive insights.

A huge thanks to Michelle Prince and everyone at Performance Publishing Group for getting this book done in minimum time and with maximum ease.

I owe much of my education as to what constitutes health and healing to people I have never met. So, a sincere thank you goes out to the pioneering doctors from the 1930s-1940s all the way through the last decade, all of whom dared to venture outside the box of traditional health care. These dedicated health practitioners desired to discover physiologies and find answers to the questions that constitute wellness and health. Their writings and discoveries continue to inspire my never-ending desire to learn and keep my resume current to the wonderful knowledge of obtaining vitality and longevity in life.

INTRODUCTION

"A healthy person has a thousand wishes,
but a sick person has only one."
Indian Proverb

Do you want to improve your overall well-being and live a longer, healthier life? Do you desire more vitality and enjoyment in your daily activities? Would you like to gain more control over your body and get that youthful feeling back? Are you looking for answers to battle the fatigue and poor health that have started creeping into your life? Are you sick and tired?

I don't know about you, but I am sick and tired!

> ... *I am sick and tired* of hearing patients come to me after being let down repeatedly by their healthcare system, a system that results in more illness than vitality and longevity.

> ... *I am sick and tired* of seeing my friends suffering with preventable diseases and dying way too young.

> ... *I am sick and tired* of giving people the answers they seek too late in their life.

> ... *I am sick and tired* of our mortality rate increasing despite medical and technological advances.

... I am sick and tired of seeing my patients being led into becoming a medical nightmare, one symptom and drug at a time, until finally they end up medicating themselves to an early grave.

We have all heard of or know of people who were diagnosed way too late in their illnesses. Recently, I saw news of Selma Blair's health struggles being highlighted everywhere, including on the cover of British *Vogue*. There she was, cane in hand, discussing how she'd suffered from an illness for several years without a diagnosis. Ultimately, she was told she had MS, but it was far too late. When I think of how much better she might have lived had she received this knowledge earlier, it pains me. Don't let that be you ... read this material and commit to creating change in your life and in those around you—starting TODAY!

Being healthy is a movement along a constant line toward health. It is a direction, not a destination or a dot on the map. It is healthy, not health. It is wellness, not well. In our journey to become healthy, we don't need to reach dire straight As Michelle Prince wrote in *Shine Through Your Story*, "No person is better than another, but some people are further along the path you may want to be on. They have much to teach. Consider these people fellow travelers on this journey called life." My hope is also that through this book, your inner spark for health and happiness becomes reignited. And I hope that spark helps you reach your potential and fulfill all that you were created to enjoy.

In your rekindled health, you will fan the flames for those around you so they may seek out their joy and happiness. You will be filled with wellness and vitality while living with your God-given inner life force. You will find fulfillment through the knowledge and power possessed in you. You will control your own life's destiny while being healthy and happy.

Life is short regardless of how long you live. So, all your time is of the essence. Why not choose to live out all of it with the best of life, for as long as possible? Live it out in radiant health, as life should be, as God had planned for you from the beginning.

Time for a New Beginning

Welcome to your personal journey towards radiant health, vitality, and longevity! By committing to focusing on what is most important in your life—your health—you can reap the benefits for the rest of your *long* life. In this book, I will share some life facts and practical tips, backed by scientific research and my own experiences, that have helped my patients fight their way back to vitality and longevity. It's time for you to stop letting everything and everyone around you keep you down!

Using the knowledge in this book and a committed attitude, you will learn to stop being the victim of the negative effects of stress and all the bad choices you made before you decided to fight for your health and well-being. Yes, the world will continue to challenge your commitment. But now you're armed with answers!

Whether you're a young adult looking to prevent chronic diseases, an aging adult wanting to reverse the effects of aging, or someone simply seeking a healthier lifestyle, this book is for you. With practical tips, scientifically backed research, and inspiring success stories, this book will motivate and empower you to take charge of your health and transform your life for the better.

Regardless of your age, the fullness of life is available to you through the secrets revealed in this book. By tapping into the 30+ years of wisdom I have accumulated as a holistic chiropractor, optimal health can be yours. All you have to do is commit to your health as a top priority and make a few simple, but effective, changes to your mindset, lifestyle, and diet. It's that easy!

It is time to begin!

How to Use This Book to Your Advantage

You did it! You have started on a new journey simply by reading this book! In terms of what you can achieve by reading this book, the sky is the limit—but you must take your time parsing through the material in here. After you read information that pertains to you, reflect on it and how you can make changes in that area. Don't just keep reading—truly *reflect*, then start incorporating small changes into your life for a big change tomorrow. You got this far, so don't stop now! Read! Reflect! Commit! Then, enjoy the riches of your efforts!

This book is not meant to be a lighthearted, easy read before bed. It is meant to be an interactive tool for you to identify where you are in life and the key areas that need your attention. Additionally, this book will provide information that will help you *prevent* illnesses you aren't even aware of yet.

As we age, things can change overnight. Many patients in their 40s tell me how they feel like they lost their eyesight overnight, and now they require reading glasses—or they have aches and pains that materialize out of nowhere. So, I would like you to at least skim areas you *think* don't pertain to you, because one day they might. Plus, if you don't recognize these issues in yourself, you may in others. By gaining knowledge of the body and how things happen, you will advance your own life and support longevity and vitality for others.

In many areas of this book, I will ask questions. These are not questions to skim by. They are meant for you to pause and reflect. The more you take time to reflect while reading this book, the better outcomes you will find when you apply the principles. Some places in the book allow lines for answering the questions, but I also recommend reading with a journal beside you. Journaling can help you look at how you've grown throughout the process.

If you don't think you have the time to really dive into the material and understand what may be holding you back, then maybe you don't have the time to find out what's plaguing your body. After all, aren't those problems what made you pick up this book in the first place?

Even so, reading is not for everyone. That's why I have also recorded some of the material in this book on my website, www. Drjoeyjones.com. Even if you've read this book, you can enjoy the little reminders in the videos. So, jump in, and let's get you on a better path to a more radiant life!

CHAPTER 1

IT'S TIME FOR CHANGE

"The greatest wealth is health."
Virgil

JUST A FEW MONTHS BEFORE this book was set to be published, an all too familiar scenario occurred. A 40-year-old male patient of mine went in to see his primary care doctor, as his insurance contract demands of him. He had to do that just so he could get a referral to see me for his low back pain and sciatica.

After his initial evaluation exam and blood work, his primary doctor recommended three different prescriptions. In the patient's history, he mentioned his stress levels and quality of sleep had worsened due to his recent economic struggles. His blood pressure was also mildly elevated at 135/90. (This could have been a side effect of white coat syndrome, traffic stressors on the way to his appointment, or caffeine consumption prior to his visit—although these factors were not discussed at the time.)

When he later received his blood work results, he was prescribed yet another medication for his cholesterol, which was 202 (only two points over the hypothetical normal). Overall, he received one prescription for anxiety and stress, one for sleep aid, one for mildly elevated blood pressure, and finally one to lower his *hypothetically* elevated cholesterol.

The concern that he expressed to me is that he is only 40 years old, and he is now on four medications that he was not on prior to that one visit to his primary care provider. Worse, that visit was supposed to be an evaluation for a referral to his chiropractor for low back pain and sciatica. Sound familiar? Again, a case of over-regulated and over-medicated.

Time to Get on Board

Riddle me this—why does it seem like everyone has catastrophic insurance coverage policies today? It's because that is all that most middle-class Americans can afford. Premiums for an affordable deductible in today's healthcare system are higher per month than most mortgage payments. So, it's time we design and sign our own patient accountability act.

If we hold others accountable for our health and health care, they will continue to let us get sicker. Then they will price us all right into Medicaid. Or they'll allow us to decline to a state of disability, only to find ourselves in Medicare or some other government program. Next thing you know, as numbers rise, they will take our qualifying factors away and we will be left without any support medically or otherwise.

If we keep going down this same road, we'll have no choice but to sign our own patient accountability act. This means that we will have to take our own responsibility for our health care. Think about that for a minute. If you lose options for quality health care, would you take better, more proactive care of your health?

Forget healthcare reform—it's time to reform your health. The best way to afford today's healthcare (Medicare included) is to need as little of it as possible. So, the train to better health—to vibrant health, and longevity with vitality, to a better life—is leaving the station! You'd better hurry up if you're going to get onboard. Because as the classic O'Jays song says, "Please don't miss this train at the station. Cause if you miss it, I feel sorry, sorry for you!"

Are you with me? If so, "Climb aboard! There are better days just ahead!"

Your Time is Now!

We're navigating a different world today than we were 100 years ago. Heck, those of us who have been around since the '60s and '70s have seen life's little pleasures escalate into life-defying decisions. Let's be real: The changes we have seen since the '80s in the nutritional depletion of our diets, the political takeover of our healthcare (or as I like to call it "sick care") system, and the publicly dysfunctional, self-preservation mentality of western society has left us stressed out, burnt out, and in dire need of enlightenment.

It is long past time to get back to the so-called "Blue Zones" mentality of living. There, we can take back control of ourselves, our children, and our loved ones with the support of our neighbors, one zip code at a time. It's time to preserve our nucleus from society's cytoplasmic toxic waste build-up, which has become the norm. Time for systemic metabolic detoxification of ourselves and society at large. Time for us to get back to "Radiant Health" for our generation and those that follow.

I know it might seem like there's a lot to process in this book. But guess what? You are *worth* the investment. And I am *worth* a lot. And we deserve to take care of our minds and bodies until we are radiating with good health. Like I always say, "It's your choice."

Think about it … if you could change one thing in your life, and that one thing was having better health, then the sky becomes the limit in terms of other benefits. Right? And if that's true, then why is your health typically not the top priority?

The older we get, the more weight we gain; the more we experience or hear of disease among friends or the death of a loved one; the more we long for our energetic days of the past; and the more we realize that our health is the most important thing there is. When you think about it, our health is the one thing that impacts all areas of our lives—either in a positive or disabling way.

This book is for the person who loves life and is in no hurry to move on to the next. The person who wants to live out this life in radiant health and vitality with their longevity. Perhaps you even want to get a step ahead? Well, if you take total control today, you'll put yourself in the driver's seat instead of the passenger's seat.

If you are still unsure whether to continue reading, below are 12 reasons you may wish to continue:

1. If looking in the mirror seems overrated to you
2. If your sleeping partner is a machine with a pump
3. If you did not have a bowel movement today
4. If your socks leave an indention 30 minutes after you take them off
5. If your beach attire *is* the cover up
6. If it takes twice as long to get half as far
7. If you feel your "get up and go" has "got up and gone"
8. If you have something on your mind, but can't remember what it is
9. If you wake up each morning just as tired as you went to bed
10. If you spend more on health care than entertainment
11. If the pharmacist knows your first name
12. If you meet your expensive (catastrophic) high-dollar deductible every year

Don't be overwhelmed by the idea that there is much you need to do or too many options. Nothing in this book is intended to be an "all or nothing" approach. You will have good days and bad days on your health journey. Don't let the bad days define what you can achieve.

That said, nothing worthwhile comes with inaction. So, the key is to *act* each and every day. If you get off track, no worries. Start again.

You need this book to commit to having, doing, and being MORE! Read this book if you are looking for that spark to reignite your flame, passion, and desire for living a long and healthy life.

This is going to be fun and liberating! Are you ready to learn more?

Your Reflection Corner

Chapter 1: It's Time for Change

Let's take a few moments to see where you are in your health journey.

- Do you feel like you've lost control of your health?
- Do you long for the good ole days when health was on your side?
- Does it take longer to heal and recover these days?
- Do you feel invigorated and ready to take charge of your day when you wake up?
- How are those bowels flowing? Are they moving every day? Could you use some help in this area?
- Are you a caretaker for someone besides yourself?
- Have you experienced a little or big trauma in your life? How have things gone for your health since then?
- Do you know there is more out of life than what you are living?
- Do you have a little or a lot of excess belly fat?
- Are you retaining water (swelling)—maybe in the face, ankles, or hands?

If you answered yes to any of these questions, this book will help!

If you have tried other avenues in the past that did not give you the results you wanted, there are new answers in this book for you to create success. When I see people fail in their efforts and give up, it's often because they can't find the right program for them. Also, they did not have the fundamental knowledge to make their program work for them because they did not know how their body works.

Do You Know?

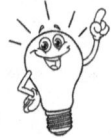

Lose Belly Tissue Following Weight Loss!

For many, this is the frustrating skin tissue that often looks like cellulite and is left behind after weight loss. This area requires a little extra patience, as these cells require longer protein absorption to rebuild lost muscle in the area. So, adequate protein ingestion and absorption is key. Again, branched-chain amino acids may be necessary to assure protein assimilation of ingested proteins.

CHAPTER 2

YOU DESERVE A RADIANT LIFE

We won't all live until we are 105—full of vitality and vigor. And we won't all be fit enough to run a 10K race at 102 years old, as Fauja Singh did in just 1 hour and 32 minutes.[1] Heck, many of us cannot even run a 10K at our current age or *any* age, let alone at 102.

Are you the one, the exception? Are you an outlier? Do you think you will beat the odds of aging?

Are you willing to do what it takes to be that person who runs a marathon or climbs a mountain in their 100s? What about your 50s? We don't all want to climb mountains or run marathons, but all of us likely want to be fit and healthy enough to *be able to* do it. This may sound a tad ambitious, but, like life itself, you've got to get it started if you're going to get it done.

No, none of us know when we will die or how it will come about. Yet there are things we can do to make the time in our bodies the best of times. Our bodies are incredible creations—far more intricate than anything science or medicine can figure out, still to this very day. Yes, a lot is known, but there is so much more that remains a mystery and a miracle. That's why it is so important to be in tune with yourself, as your health care practitioner does not always know what is best. We must honor our bodies the same way we would honor any miracle of life.

---

[1]   9 Oldest Marathon Runners in The World - Oldest.org

*"What? Know ye not that your body is the
temple of the Holy Ghost which is in you, which
ye have of God, and ye are not your own?"*
1 Corinthians 6:19 (KJV)

Yes, you read that right. Your body is a temple and should be honored. After all, you only get one body in your life. It's like a car—based on how hard you drive it, how you maintain it, and how you treat it, it may wear out faster than others. And you can learn to maximize its full potential.

We cannot live our lives "hoping" that we don't get sick or that we will stay physically able and mentally sound forever. Without deliberate efforts to maintain proper nutrition and stay physically active, we will become one of the statistics we so often read about: early death, premature aging, comorbidities, loss of enjoyment in living, and more.

As we age, we think, "That will never happen to me." Or worse, we think, "I expect this to happen to me at some point because of my genes." What story are you telling yourself about your health and your potential for longevity and vitality? Are you taking steps now so that you don't find yourself consumed by disease in the future? Do you have control over your health, or is it an afterthought? Or have you handed over your health to others to tell you how to manage it?

As we get older, we need to take off our blinders and realize that the worst can happen to us all—unless we take proactive steps to ensure our best outcomes. Not only do we need to take deliberate steps to ensure our best outcomes, but these steps also must be specific to our age and according to our current health considerations. We are all designed to uniquely live out our own individualized lives, so we cannot fit into any cookie cutter approach. There are so many books out there that don't take the personal experience into account. That's why I am trying to educate my readers about what good health is and that longevity and vitality are possible—so you can take this knowledge and extend your life.

More than anything, you need to have a vision for yourself. You must *want* more, no matter where your starting place is in life. Later in the book, we will work together to create your vision (i.e., your dream future), the goals to support your vision, and the activities to support your goals. In doing so, you WILL achieve your vision. Without knowledge, direction, and action in your life, you will likely never achieve your dreams. In the end, it is up to you to be accountable for truly living your life, rather than sleepwalking through it.

Aging should be a cherished experience—one earned and well-deserved. You must dive into life, rather than living like some version of the walking dead. When you are fit for life, you can age and eventually die healthy. And isn't that what we all want? To die healthy, vibrant, and fit in our old, old age. In fact, I hear too many people say they don't want to live until they are old because they don't want to live without vitality. To live an old and healthy life, you need knowledge, because knowledge at any age is power! My passion is to empower you so that you are not reliant on others' opinions and experiences.

As a Doctor of Chiropractic for my entire adult career, it has been my mission to improve the quality of human life. I understand not only that it is important for me to do my part, but also that I have a burning desire to educate my patients on preventative care and how they can be their own champion of health. Too often, I see patients who are deep into a health crisis. I want to turn the tide; I want to see my patients avoid health crises altogether and be a health statistic of vitality and longevity.

See, I have the knowledge you need after focusing on health, wellness, and vitality for over 30 years. I feel like I have seen it all—or at least everything out there to date. Few things surprise me anymore. All the troubled souls that walk through my door find hope and answers. I want the same for you, which is why I am writing this book to reach the masses! I wish I could help every person on this earth, but until then, I will touch everyone I can through my books, teachings, and practice.

When you have knowledge about your body and how it works, you can set yourself up for long-term great health. When we have good health, the advantages are endless. My patients have increased confidence as a result of taking control of their bodies and health, which creates more opportunities in their lives for happiness and vitality. And when they are happier, everyone they touch is impacted positively through their example. The possibilities are endless!

Down Under

I like to look at the whole patient, not just the one area that is bothering you. I dive deep and get to know what the causes are, the history of how you got to where you are, and how everything and everyone around you feeds your issues. As you go through this book, I would encourage you to do the same for yourself. Don't just focus on your problem area—focus on advancing yourself all around and proactively.

In my program, I understand that the patient is only one part of the equation back to wellness, vitality, and longevity. The environment surrounding my patients/clients is a huge contributing factor. To find good health, we must look at our overall well-being and environment.

I want more for you than good health and vitality for the long haul. I want that to be the springboard into a better life altogether. I want radiance and prosperity in your future—all around! The four keys I have found in unlocking the power of a happy, healthy, prosperous life include:

1. Support – helping others have what they want and need: their health
2. Encouragement – helping empower others with the knowledge to improve their quality of life
3. Accountability – helping others become the person in charge to become the person they want, need, and deserve to be
4. Faith – helping others strengthen their belief in a larger purpose and giving them knowledge so they know they are not alone

Most people want to have more control of their lives but don't know where to start. Or they feel overwhelmed with information and options. Then there are others who have the desire to get more control over their health, but they struggle with self-control. Lastly, there are people who have lost hope that they can reverse their path to increased ailments. They believe that getting older is just a natural part of life. Well, to you, wherever you are in your journey, the material in this book can help you in your endeavor to obtain vitality with longevity!

Turn Back the Hands of Time

Would you like to turn back the hands of time on your health, wellness, and vitality? Are you ready for a change? Let's look at a few areas where this book can help you get on that exact track to reversing or preventing damage. Do any of these statements below sound like you?

- I *wish* I could reverse the damage I have done to myself!
- I *wish* I could get out from under the mounds of medications controlling my existence.
- I *wish* I was thriving and loving life instead of just getting by and surviving.
- I *wish* I could keep up with my schedule.

We cannot depend on a *wish* for a radiant life full of vitality and vigor. I have had so many patients come to me with regret, sharing that they *wish* they had paid closer attention to their health over the years. They did not know they would face so many health hurdles so quickly, so they did not take the best care of themselves.

Countless times, patients return to me emphasizing how they *wish* they had acted on my previous suggestions, and now they need a refresher on what to do. This time, the questions asked are a lot different. They have further to come back from and the pathway back to where they intended is even harder.

It is never too late, but the earlier you start, the better! I have one 75-year-old friend who has told me that she feels better now than she did in her 50s. This too can be you, no matter the age. It is the same for me, too. I have been down this path (more later on my story). If I can do it, you can too!

> *"So, teach us to number our days, that we*
> *may apply our hearts unto wisdom."*
> Psalm 90:12 KJV

Life is unpredictable. Yes, our days are numbered, but just how many days we have left remains a mystery. We must plan for setbacks and do more than hope for the best! We cannot wait to make a change "when" we reach a certain age. We don't need to keep changing our to-do lists, eliminating things we no longer can do. Prevention is key—and knowledge is the key to prevention!

Doesn't gaining your power back sound great? When I talk about power, I am referring to the power to regain youthful vitality, energy, and the zest for life. I am not going to do anything "for" you. You will be in the driver's seat of your own health, vitality, and longevity from here on out. Now is where *you* turn back the hands of time and discover more radiance in your life.

Turn the Page on Your Health and Longevity ...

This book has been inside of me forever, *begging* to be released. I just could not wait another moment, because I know people needed to hear these words. Just yesterday, I was talking to one patient about this book, and she broke down crying. She told me that she needs the book NOW!

She told me how she feels so strong when I talk with her and that she knows how to stay on track whenever she leaves my office. Then, she gets home and loses her attention. Soon, she finds herself off her wellness track. She begged me to hurry up and finish writing this book so she can have it with her when the times get tough and her commitment wavers. She wants to get back to being the star in her own movie, and she knows that this book will help her do exactly that.

Stand Up and Stretch!

Yes, I said stand up and STRETCH! As you stretch your body, ask yourself what is burning to be released within you? What is your burning passion and drive asking of you? To achieve any dream or goal, you need your mind, body, and soul to be fit. The great Muhammad Ali once said something along the lines of, "The secret to achieving your dreams, is to first wake up." If you have a big dream, it won't mean much if you don't have the energy and vitality left to enjoy or maintain it. I am here to help!

Information vs. Misinformation

I have a burning passion to ring the alarm bells as loudly as possible, because everyone needs to know what is happening to their health. There is so much misinformation out there—information that addresses symptoms and nothing else. Too often, misinformation is given to patients that disempowers them, as it doesn't allow them to address underlying health concerns. Without answers, many give up and resolve to live with the discomfort, pain, and tiredness. Too few keep searching for possible answers, alternatives, and opportunities.

Be the exception. Don't give up on yourself just yet—no matter what you hear from the experts! Too many people give up after hearing their doctor tell them there is little hope or possibility outside of regulating and medicating. Or these doctors emphasize excuses such as "well, you're just getting older," and tell their patients they may just have to live without ever feeling normal again. The best outcomes happen before people are in a medical nightmare. A medical nightmare includes taking multiple medications, having multiple diagnosis, having multiple surgeries, having chronic debilitating symptoms, incurring high yearly medical expenses, and/or having a poor prognosis for recovery. Don't let medical nightmares rule your future life!

As patients/clients enter my office, they are treated as the most valuable resource in the world, not just another number for the day. Do you treat yourself as invaluable? Does your doctor? Does your schedule reflect your health goals? Are you a priority in your life?

Are you setting yourself up for success or failure? Your schedule reflects the value you are placing on your health and your life. How does your schedule mimic the desired life you want to achieve? Yes, that's right. We have some work to do—on your schedule and your life!

In my office, we supply people with information to empower them to find the right answers for their health. Life is different for my patients because I desire to provide them with real answers. I don't just pacify them by addressing symptoms and giving them excuses. Instead, we work *together* to address the core problems causing their pain and inability to thrive. By educating and empowering them, we create change together!

Who Do You Place Your Trust in Regarding Your Health?

More and more these days, patients are looking to alternatives in their medical care. It is my life's mission to help people discover, and sometimes re-discover, the secrets to good health and ultimate fulfillment. I help my patients regain control over their health by diving into what led them to their current state of health. I help them investigate past decisions, traumas, and their environment to see what is holding their health hostage. It's so sad to me that people are being misguided when it comes to their options to better health.

Too often, I see people having placed faith in their doctor's less-than-positive outcomes, only to find that there are so many other pathways to free themselves from illness. So, my goal is to push you to empower yourself. You should not take what anyone tells you about your health as the only truth. As President Reagan once said, "Trust, but verify." Information is out there, but you must find it or find someone who really has your best interest in their heart to help.

It is a sad truth that doctors are being backed into corners in how they can treat people. Remember, doctors are supposed to be healers, and many do good work. But there are so many rules and requirements that back them into a corner for treating in ways that are against their own instincts and knowledge. And for many other doctors, providing health care is just a means of income.

Doctors today just don't have the ability to give individualized treatment as much as doctors of the past. On top of that, there are so many financial considerations that get in the way of the decision-making process for treatment options. Don't get me wrong—there are *definitely* good reasons for protocols and guidelines. But when you get too many, it comes at the expense of the patient rather than the benefit.

It is my mission to stop having patients come in after years of searching for a diagnosis, get a diagnosis, and then never hear any other options. They are told there is only a protocol for symptom suppression to treat their condition. This scenario plays out in my office time and time again. Patients are without relief, so they look for alternative ways to treat themselves beyond an overflowing medicine cabinet. They feel confused, overwhelmed, and out of control.

Again, when patients troubled by their health work with me, I address them by looking at the whole person. I don't just look at what is in front of me or what they decided to share with me. I don't just look at a specific area, but rather at a person as a whole. I get that God made your body to heal itself, so I work with your body's healing processes to bring out better outcomes by partnering with, instead of destroying, your own body's innate healing power.

There are so many symptoms that people forget or don't consider as anything more than "aging less gracefully." Oh, and there are those symptoms that people are too shy to share or too hesitant to present. Good news: I have an in-depth questionnaire that gives people a chance to present their symptoms in a private way. This way, things that go under the radar of a patient are discovered by a thoughtful review of the whole body. Let me tell you now, in my office, you are more than your symptoms!

When we talk about being healthy, there is always so much more under the surface. Someone may think that they or someone they know is healthy—right up until the moment they have a heart attack. Take, for example, the seasoned competitive marathon runner who heads out one morning for his daily five-mile run and has a massive heart attack in his front yard at age 40. Was he fit? Most people would agree, yes, he was. But was he healthy? Maybe not so much.

Then there is someone like Winston Churchill. He was overweight, smoked, and drank throughout the day. He was probably not a poster child for being healthy and fit. And yet, Mr. Churchill lived into his 90s. Could we say he was healthier than the marathon runner who died 50 years younger?

This is proof that you cannot just look at someone and know if they are healthy or not. You must look at more than their psychical appearance. As a doctor, I am often able to identify warning signs from the outside, but I cannot see everything under the surface. **I stress to my patients, "Don't get fit to become healthy, be healthy to become fit."**

It is time to experience the radiant life you deserve—for the long haul! I want to see you out there in life looking radiant and living actively into your 100s! I want those people who are 10 and 20 years younger than you to look at you, green with envy for all your energy and vitality, and think, "How does he/she do it?"

I want you to be a shining, glorious example to others. I want to show you all that is possible, so you can spread the word. Are you ready to create more vitality and impact in this world? Let's begin!

Your Reflection Corner

Chapter 2: You Deserve a Radiant Life

It's time to reflect on what is holding you back from a radiant life and a full commitment to change! A radiant life will not look the same person to person, so let's figure out what it looks like to you.

Your Definition of a Radiant Life:

- What would a more radiant life mean to you?
- Do you want it?
- How badly?
- Why?
- Are you ready to go after it?

If the thought of taking more control over your health and life is making you stressed or fearful of exhaustion, know that there is more to life than what you're experiencing today. Let's check in with ourselves for a moment.

Activity:

- Think about what is important to you ... mentally, physically, spiritually, and emotionally. Now, rate yourself on a scale of 1-10 depending on where you are in relation to where you want to be in those four areas.
- Do you have a quality of life that makes you proud?
- If you don't make any changes in the next year, three years, or five years, what will happen to your current quality of life?
- Are you at a crossroads?
- Are you conquering life or is it conquering you?

Pop Quiz: What is one thing you can do starting today that can impact every area of your life?

The answer? Start focusing on your health! Trust me, it will pay dividends immediately. Even if you take baby steps like the following, you will start to feel the difference:

- Stop eating those inflammatory foods (breads, grains) and exchange them with quality proteins, small apples, or some lightly salted pecans.
- Get off the couch (or office chair) and dance around for five minutes every hour.
- Drink one glass of extra water today or drink a glass of water between any drinks that are not water.
- Wake up with a little mild stretching. Give yourself a hug, roll that head of yours around, and try to touch your feet.
- Start the day with three deep breaths—hold them for a few seconds, then exhale long and slow.
- Eat five small meals a day, starting with eating a breakfast fit for kings and queens.
- Add a positive self-affirmation to each day. Something like, "Today, I move forward in life."

Yes, we are going to go big on some changes suggested in the following pages—but don't forget that you have got to where you are today making one decision, one day at a time. Sometimes, you just need to move slowly and patiently. Small changes can have a big impact, if you stay consistent.

And remember: Do what suits you best. Whatever strategy you feel makes you most successful in the long haul, employ it. The goal is to create change but have fun with how you do it.

Consistency is key, though. Make sure you stay consistent with your plan if you want to see results!

Do You Know?

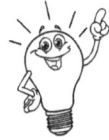

Collagen and the Skin

Collagen supplementation is a great way to improve skin tone and elasticity. Personally, I prefer plant-based collagen products to marine-based ones. Collagen-based protein formulas can be difficult to absorb and stressful to some digestive tracts. I recommend including digestive enzymes and a complete branched-chain amino acid supplement to improve absorption and assimilation.

CHAPTER 3

How Did I Get Here?

*The road to ill health is not paved with good
intentions. It is paved with the lack of attention.*

FIRST THING'S FIRST: DON'T BE so hard on yourself! You have been
doing the best you can with what you know and the tools you have!
Yes, you can do more. Yes, you will do more! But first you need the
knowledge necessary to take back control of your life. We usually
know better than to make poor lifestyle choices, but somehow, we
go into survival mode, and the poor decisions come naturally to us.
Before we know it, we are sick, tired, over- or underweight, suffering
from disease, and more.

Sound familiar?

We often push ourselves so hard with our family and career that
we neglect our body and health until we cannot ignore the warning
signs any longer. We find that we are either burning the candle at both
ends or have become a little too comfortable on the couch. Either
way, our way of living becomes a danger to our health and long-term
happiness. As we become restricted in our lives, neglecting to take
care of our bodies and mind, we set ourselves up for failure and loss!

As we stop investing and start ignoring our own needs, we
inevitably shorten our own vitality, and possibly even our lifespan.
When we do so, we are also taking from the life of those we love—
because by allowing ourselves to stay down and depleted, our loved
ones suffer from our attitudes and health!

When life takes over and we lose control, it takes a toll, often blindsiding us. This can happen slowly over time, until one day it finally hits us! We start recognizing that things don't feel like they used to, and we cannot do the things we could do in the past so easily these days. In other cases, it may happen in an instant through a life-changing event such as a heart attack or stroke.

We can suffer a trauma that impedes our focus on ourselves—maybe through a loss, like the loss of a job, loved one, divorce, or through illness. We could also find ourselves in a caretaker situation overnight, leaving little or no energy to care for ourselves at the end of the day. It may even be a "freak accident" that, in an instant, changed our life forever.

Regardless of how we got here, the path in front of us can look the same, at least to some degree. Many of us find ourselves stuck in a sort of "Groundhog Day," where we truly stop living. We just go through the motions. Others may be more proactive and try to find ways to make the most of it, but the crushing weight of our burdens can keep us down.

Once we get to this place of feeling unhealthy, defeated, unhappy, and weak, we start buying into the idea of aging and that it is outside of our control. We let ourselves go—often because of our own neglect. This is when things spiral out of control.

… I want to feel better, but I am just so tired!

… I want more for my life, but I just don't have time to make changes!

… What happened to me? Where did my vitality go?

… I am so embarrassed that I got here. When I was young, I told myself I would never allow myself to look or be like the person I have become. All I do is hide from pictures and hide at home to avoid people seeing me like this.

... I don't want to buy clothes anymore, so I wear the same ones, day in and day out. These are not attractive clothes, but I feel like they help hide my shame.

... I never thought I would live this long. If I had, I would have paid more attention to my body and health.

Have any of these thoughts been in your head at some point in time ... maybe as you looked into the mirror this morning? Alternatively, have you been telling yourself any of the following:

... Fitness is for other people. My achy body cannot do it anymore!

... I'm just too old! It's too late to get my health back.

... It's just my genetics! There is nothing I can do.

... It's all just too much! I don't know where to start.

... There is no hope! I've tried everything!

... Health is too complicated. I don't understand all the rules! It's just too much!

... Nothing works for me! I give up!

... But my doctor said no solution exists and that I must get comfortable with feeling bad every day!

I know it may not feel like it from where your mind is today, but I am here to tell you there is a way out! There is a pathway to vitality and longevity at any age.

Are you still not convinced? Are you still doubtful—feeling confused, frustrated, or hopeless? Do you think you have too far to go and feel like you'll never make it to the finish line? Do you want more out of your days?

Well, guess what? You can have it! Trust me! There are answers— YES, even for you, no matter your starting place!

I know you can achieve more for your health and vitality because I have taken many of my patients/clients through this exact transformation. Nothing is better to me than witnessing my clients and patients turn their discouragement into confidence. I have helped many from all walks of life and starting points, but I see the best results in those who are proactively replenishing and renewing themselves before the RED warning light starts flashing.

> *"Although the Lord gives you the bread of adversity*
> *and the water of affliction, your teachers will be hidden*
> *no more; with your own eyes you will see them."*
> Isaiah 30:20 (NIV)

Do you love yourself enough to do whatever is required to live the life intended for you? I want you to take a chance and walk with me. Take the energy you spend on judging yourself and turning down your invitations and refocus it on creating a more bountiful life. You are not alone. I am here to help!

First, let's rewind a bit and figure out why our bodies were created. After that, we'll delve into how you got *here*, to this point where you decided to say, "No more!" I am so excited for you, because I can see your light coming more into focus—a light of joy, peace, vitality, and longevity.

Your Starting Point ... Why Were You Created?

Remember when you had all the answers as a still-budding adult? You were at your peak of health and vitality, without an aching bone or muscle. There was little you could not do with your body, and your metabolism was running like a well-oiled machine. What happened? Is that all there is for your vitality?

Yes, remember when you were young and knew that you would never let yourself go like all those you saw growing old far before their time? So, how did this happen to you? Is this all there is for your life—aches, tiredness, and depression, all without confidence? I say NO!

> *"Marvelous are thy works, and the*
> *soul knoweth right well."*
> Psalms 139:14 (NIV)

We were born with all we needed within us to sustain a long life full of vitality and good health. OK, you may have been burdened with a few things that you had no control over. Even so, you were created so that you could prosper and grow. You were given the building blocks for success just where you are today. But there is *more*. Let's unpack it.

The Power Within

You have more power available to you than you admit to yourself! All of mother nature's creatures are designed to fully flourish before they die.

Our bodies are powerful machines. They know what they need and when they need it. The intricacies within allow our bodies to talk to us—when we are hungry, tired, thirsty. Whatever it may be, our bodies are always talking to us. The aches could just mean we need to stretch. The headaches could be a signal that we need more water. Our lack of energy is likely a sign that we need to do more, not less. Our sleepless nights may be telling us that we need to make changes in our lives due to high stress or nutritional deficiencies.

Our bodies are talking to us all the time. We may just be treating our bodies like our longtime spouse, tuning them out when we don't care what they have to say or because we've already heard it. By learning to take time and listen to our bodies, we can find our way back to better health. Even if this is the only thing you get out of this book, I will be happy for you!

If you are reconsidering your choice to read this book and give yourself a shot at a better life, I am here to tell you that you were created to live a prosperous life and grow within yourself. You were not created to be stagnant or let the enemy steal your days from you. No, this is not a book on religion, but we must honor our God, our Creator, for His amazing masterpiece He created: us. I mean, how can we talk about the body and how it works without giving a shoutout to our Creator. He formed us, and He provides and nourishes us as we breathe, eat, and drink throughout our days.

Without giving our Creator credit for the intricacies of how our bodies are made to heal themselves, then we are on our own. Trust me, a path alone will be very lonely and is the path of depletion, not increase and renewal. By leaning into our God-given purpose for living, we can find comfort that we have been created for perfection, not destruction. Remember this, "Your body is always seeking wellness and radiant health even when you are not."

You Are Worthy!

Life is meant to be full of excitement and wonder! Our days are meant for joy, peace, and feeling ALIVE! Do you feel ALIVE in life? Or are you just counting down the moments? Are you living life passionately?

I am here to tell you that, no matter where you are in life, there is MORE! You are here because there is something more you are supposed to experience or achieve. To do so, we must show up as our best! Are you showing up as your best, day in and day out? If the answer is no, no worries. That's what this book is here for.

The book of Thomas tells us, "If you bring forth what is in you, what you have will save you." How exciting is that? Yes, through our faith, we can see the bigger picture for ourselves and how the nourishment of our body is critical to achieve our vision. We must take what we have and build it up, not tear it down through bad habits and self-abusive tendencies. We have a lot more control than we give ourselves credit for.

If you doubt that you are worthy of the investment and having more in life, lean on God's word.

"So, God created mankind in his own image, in the image of God he created him; male and female he created them."
Genesis 1:27 (NIV)

"For we are God's handiwork, created in Christ Jesus to do good works, which God prepared in advance for us to do."
Ephesians 2:10 (NIV)

"You therefore must be perfect, as your heavenly Father is perfect."
Matthew 5:48 (ESV)

How Did You Get Here?

We all have seen better times in our lives—times we felt more in control, times we were at peace with ourselves, times when the possibilities in our lives seemed endless, and times when we were bursting with joy in our everyday lives, truly feeling alive. Remember those days? Maybe you are there now. If so, I applaud you.

By looking at how you got here, you can figure out how to unwind where you are and ultimately take back your health and vitality. I know all the information can be overwhelming sometimes, but I am here to walk you through it in bite-sized pieces.

I believe in you! Do you? Do you believe that you can have more, be more, do more, and experience all other kinds of more? If you don't believe, no worries. I will give you the knowledge to boost your confidence and get your mojo back. The belief in us starts with the mind.

It is not all on us. There are so many things working against us that need awareness too. Just take the advice of Marcia Angell, American physician and author, who once said, "Over the past two decades the pharmaceutical industry has moved very far from its original high purpose of discovering and producing useful drugs. Now (it's) primarily a marketing machine to sell drugs of dubious benefit."

The Art of Aging

Your chronological age (calculated in terms of the passage of time) and your biological age (related to biology or living organisms) do not have to occur at the same rate. The secret to slowing down our biological aging—the aging of our bodies—is to control our metabolism and inflammation. And when we look at what is causing our metabolism and inflammation to go bonkers, we first must look at blood sugar levels. There are tons of books that discuss the detrimental impacts of sugar on our lives and our health.

The single greatest way to keep inflammation in check is to maintain healthy blood sugar levels. And if you want to keep your blood sugar in check, you must start by reducing your carbohydrate intake. I know, ladies, you love, love, love your carbohydrates. But I am here to tell you that if you love yourself, then you need to get a new relationship with carbohydrates—one less romanticized by how they make you feel! Yes, they can feel good to eat, but they wreak havoc on your insides.

Processed foods, wheat, grains, flour, sugar, and artificial sweeteners are devilish to your system! Yes, when I talk about carbohydrates, I am especially referring to processed foods, wheat, grains, milled flour, sugar, and artificial sweeteners. And yes, I took the time to repeat the list so all those foods will be engrained in your mind.

From a technical perspective, the reason you need to find an exit door for these foods in your diet is because they trigger a reaction called *glycation*—the biological process where sugar binds to a protein and certain fats. This results in deformed, poorly-functioning molecules. These sugar proteins are so damaging to our bodies. They are technically called advanced glycation end products (or AGEs—which just so happens to spell exactly what these proteins do to our bodies).

These AGEs are precursors to diseases such as obesity, diabetes, Alzheimer's (now being called type III diabetes), cardiovascular disease, ADD, ADHD, and so many (if not most) autonomic disorders that are on the rise today. Even stress and depression fit right in with other inflammatory disorders, as they tend to have higher levels of inflammatory blood markers and shorter telomeres (for more info, see the section on recommended blood panels).

It is critical to reduce your risk of developing these disabling degenerative disorders. They are not only extremely costly to you but are also costly to both our society and healthcare system—better known as our "sick care system" (which is the single greatest contributor to sky-high costs in America for health care). There are answers, and I am here to help you find them.

If you start today, you can get on the right track to better health and vitality by reducing your glucose levels close to or below 80. Glucose levels that stay elevated at 90 or higher will eventually lead to sugar handling issues. You will be set up for bigger problems down the road like insulin resistance, type II diabetes, pre-diabetes, advanced rate of aging, shortened life span, and a whole host of other diseases.

If you get nothing else out of this book, at least get this: Every time you allow processed foods, wheat, grains, and artificial sweeteners to cross your mouth, you are reducing your life expectancy—along with the quality of life for the time you have left. I only hope that from this moment on, you at least ask yourself, "Are there other options geared towards my body's desired nutritional needs—perhaps a healthy fat, protein, or fruit?"

You may say that you have already tried and failed, but that is why you are here: to get answers and different perspectives, and to create a pathway to better health and longevity. The answers of the past were likely preached to you. Now, you are going to learn the knowledge in this book and develop your own pathway. By taking control of your health, you will be able to devise a unique plan according to your likes, lifestyle, and more.

Average Life Expectancy is Decreasing

According to the CDC's website, life expectancy in the US fell in 2021 for the second year in a row. It was the first time that it had fallen for two consecutive years in over 100 years. The CDC states that the average life span in my state of Alabama is 73, which is unacceptable. Your 70s are your golden years—time to shine, not fade into the shadows of life!

What I have found in my practice is that the average prescription medicine consumption for a typical 40-year-old is four, 50-year-old is five, 60-year-old is six, and 70-year-old is seven. As I have explained to them, what you will not see is a 90-year-old taking nine … because their life will have already expired. I honestly cannot remember a 90-year-old in my clinic, or family history, taking more than one, maybe two, prescriptions. Even then, those prescriptions are usually for something mild like a diuretic for blood pressure. Surviving in your seventh or eighth decade medicated and regulated is not living—it's surviving without thriving.

When someone says they don't want to live to 90 or beyond, it's because they fear getting older. They fear living a life with a long, drawn-out disease and the unnecessary complications linked to it, such as heart and/or respiratory issues, arthritic conditions (like body and joint pain), and loss of memory and mind. Sadly, this scenario seems to be becoming more the norm. But you shouldn't fear growing old. To quote Lao Tzu, "Must I fear what others fear? What nonsense!"

Aging should not be a demise, but rather a cherished experience, one earned and well deserved. News flash: When you are fit for life, you can age and eventually die healthy. It's OK. You don't have to die sick or diseased, hooked up to life-prolonging machines, void of both your dignity and life quality. Start seeking out the answers to longevity and vitality earlier in life, even in your 20s and 30s.

But if those days are already behind you, that is OK too. Knowledge, at any age, is power. With power comes control, and with control comes confidence. And in tandem, these three powers give you control over life's stresses.

Sadly, most health care today is profit driven. Practitioners are highly stressed to produce numbers and create volume for their corporate entities. Little time is spent knowing the patient, including their lifestyle, stressors, and other underlying conditions that may be driving abnormal—or should I say pre-determined—or normal ranges. For example, a normal blood pressure range is 120/80 mmHg, whereas cholesterol is 200 mg/dL. But depending on patient specifics, the "normal" ranges may not be the optimal range. Our healthcare system is not driven by successful clinical outcomes— or by positive doctors' results, for that matter. It is driven by the financial success of corporate America's bottom line. It is a broken system; it is toxic and in dire need of humanitarian change, but I wouldn't hold my breath for that!

It is your God-given right to control your own health, your life, and how you choose your journey. Vitality and longevity are yours for the taking, but you must *take them*!

Giving sole responsibility of your health to another—including a healthcare system focused on sick care and profit-driven corporations—could put you in with the average medicated numbers for your chronological age group, as mentioned earlier. Statistically speaking, medicating your way through life will greatly reduce your chances for vitality further down the road. It is not as if society's corporate-driven healthcare, by the likes of Big Pharma and the Food Commerce, is out to diminish your quality of life. It is about profit—that is their bottom line. If one gets hurt along the way, it's only collateral damage.

Blame and Responsibility

We all wish to be more responsible for our own quality of health. That is, we wish to have the ability to respond with awareness to the circumstances affecting our health rather than react to the consequences of our actions. We want to be authoritative, empowered in our own health: to be in charge and able to make the genuine decisions that affect us. There can be no true responsibility without awareness, and no accountability without control.

One of the weaknesses of the western medical approach is that we have made the physician the only authority and the patient all too often the mere recipient of a treatment, cure, or outcome. Thus, people are deprived of the opportunity to become responsible for their outcomes. None of us are necessarily to be blamed if we succumb to illness or death. That possibility is there for any of us at any given time. However, the more we can come to learn about ourselves (for example, the effects of diets, lifestyle choices, stresses, etc.), the less prone we are to become passive victims.

The mind and body links must be seen not only for our understanding of illness, but also for our comprehension of health. In health and healing, every piece of information, every bit of truth is imperative. If a link exists between one's emotions, lifestyle, diet, and physiology, not to educate them of such an existence may very well deprive them of a powerful tool in their quest for longevity with radiant health.

My years in practice have helped me identify three major contributing factors predisposing our health to life's unwanted stressors. The three factors include a lack of information, uncertainty, and loss of control. Yes, there is information out there, but far often too much of it. Or it is too hard to employ into our lives, or it does not fit our needs exactly.

When we think of loss of control, we cannot ignore the impact that society has on our health. The new generation wants to be influencers, but I say we are all influencers and consumers. I want you to learn how to consume knowledge that supports your health and doesn't take you further from it. I also want you to consume information, but then keep searching for more and more until it all fits together. (See my recommended reading section for more resources and ideas.)

Most societal-related health problems are not public health problems at all instead, they are the result of millions upon millions of individually responsible decisions, lifestyle choices, and self-imposed afflictions and diseases. They are also exacerbated by our social, political, and economic environments.

Your Story

There is nothing more powerful in your life than your story—the one you tell yourself, the story others tell you. It's not just the big events in life that change you, but those little things you experience over many years or repeatedly. Those moments can alter how you experience the world and your life.

When I first meet a patient, I like to really understand who they are and what they have been through. It is so important to figure out what led them to this place of disease or discomfort. There is always a story behind it. And almost always, the story starts in the early years, back when we were trying to figure out who we are and what was happening to us.

Some patients have tools and support systems to pull them through mostly unscathed during the tough times, but many still find themselves suffering in silence. At an early age, we are taught not to cry, not to show emotion. This approach does not make us stronger, and sometimes it expands our experience across years rather than just a few moments of grief. We become fragile or hard and distrustful. All the while, our health is suffering.

The toxicity from these moments starts stirring within us. Our gut gets its first punch and may not heal for many years—in fact, it may never heal. The burdens of our everyday lives seem to weigh us down beyond our strength. We lose ourselves. We use all our energy just to go through the day, never finding joy.

If this sounds like you, there is help out there for you. There are so many resources. First, you must work through your trauma immediately—be it physical or psychological—and as you do, your health will start to return. Don't go it alone, though. There are trained professionals to give you support for healing your mental health, and there are life and health coaches like me who can help you get back your vitality, hope, joy, and peace, primarily through better nutrition and fitness.

There is a way forward for you no matter where you are. I am here to serve. A burning passion to serve has been placed in my heart, and that includes serving you. I hope you find your answers in the coming chapters, but if you feel you need more or have a unique situation, I am still here to work with you to find your answers. All you have to do is contact me through my website, www.drjoeyjones.com.

You are not the exception, and you are meant for a great and powerful life. That life can start today. Let's start the walk toward more! As Seneca the Younger once said, "My joy in learning is partly that it puts me in a position to teach."

Before We Start

Before we get started on our mission, we need to get out of our heads and into our bodies. Far too often, we dismiss the minor inconveniences in our day that result from our poor health. For instance, we may be a little constipated, but we blow it off with our own diagnosis of too much cheese. Yes, diet can impact your bowels, but there are so many little symptoms that we brush off as nothing or as part of getting older when they *really* might signal a bigger issue.

As you educate yourself with this book, pay special attention to what your body is saying. For instance, being tired is not the only state your body may be in, no matter how busy you are at work. So many mothers come into my office thinking that tiredness is just a part of motherhood. Yes, there are tiring days (and even months with a newborn), but you should not have a tiring *life*. If this is you, there are answers!

Don't accept little nuisance symptoms as "just life" or part of getting older. Being moody, experiencing forgetfulness, combating leaky urination, feeling blah, carrying excess belly fat, and other symptoms are not normal! As we get older or more advanced with health issues, we often get used to pain and discomfort—so much so that we forget about them. We just accept them and do nothing to cure them or prevent them from worsening.

Get intimate with your body and its signals. I want you to have a deeper focus on your body and how it is working for you. As you become more aware and start to identify symptoms that relate to your body, write them down. The symptoms are clues to your bigger picture of health. For instance, some of us have an eye that has been twitching off and on for years, so you don't even think about it anymore. There is something you can do to get that to go away for good!

As you move through this book, there are answers. Yes, the biggest impact you can make on your future is preventative care. Sometimes, just building up your building blocks of good health can be enough. But other times, your body needs more to become whole.

Your Reflection Corner

Chapter 3: How Did I Get Here?

When you look in the mirror, do you hear your thoughts saying:

- This is not who I am. I don't know the person reflected in the mirror.
- How did I get here?
- I need a change in my life!
- I cannot do "this" anymore.
- I want my old self back!

Now, let's assess your current health:

- Do you feel winded when you walk around the block?
- Is your waist circumference increasing year by year?
- Do you feel tired when you wake up?
- Do you feel overwhelmed before you begin?
- Are you experiencing bowel movements daily?
- Do you require sleep aids to sleep?

Our lives can change over time, but they can also change in a moment.

- Did you have a life event or trauma period you can identify from your past?
    - What was that traumatic event or time period?
    - How did you respond to it?
    - How did your body respond to it?

- If you cannot think of a traumatic event in your life, tell me, what was going on with you in the weeks, months, and years leading up to your decline in health?
- Unlocking the events in our lives and how we reacted to them can give us clues as to what toxins we may still be holding

onto ... especially those dark moments that we keep buried. So, please don't skip over this area too quickly. It really does hold a big piece of your puzzle!

What are your health goals?

What do you feel is standing in the way of your health goals?

How would you rank the following on a scale of 1-10:

- Overall health: _____
- Support system: _____
- Willingness to create changes in your life: _____
- Ability to visualize yourself achieving your health goals: _____
- Friendship with yourself as you look in the mirror (i.e., self-talk): _____
- Accountability environment: _____

- Reliance on faith: _____
- Encouragement environment: _____
- Belief in yourself (i.e., confidence): _____
- Belief you can do and be more: _____

What do the above rankings tell you about your ability to create positive change and achieve your goals? If you see an area where you rank particularly low, highlight it with a highlighter so you can more clearly identify what is holding you back. Is it the same as you stated in the question above?

Now that you know your "how you got here," it will be easier to get where you want to go. Your limitations within are exposed, so what are you going to do about them?

....

....

....

....

....

....

....

Do You Know?

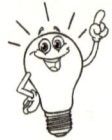

Incontinence and the Whole Food B Vitamin Connection

One of my most successful treatment protocols for bladder incontinence when associated with muscular weakness of the supporting bladder and pelvic muscles is whole food vitamin B supplementation, along with Kegel exercises. One of the major causes for B vitamin deficiencies in our diets today is processed bread consumption. Does anybody you know eat a ton of processed bread?

Processed bread consumption leaches B vitamin reserves from our bodies, resulting in loss of muscular tone and nerve conduction strength (which leads to bladder incontinence). Resupplying these B vitamin reserves improves muscle function, thus addressing the cause and ultimately reducing the effect. FYI: Synthetic multi-B vitamin complexes are not effective.

Chapter 4

What Has Happened and Is Happening to Me?

Are you tired of being tired?

Are you sick of being sick?

Have you woken up to one too many "wake up calls" from your health?

When we feel sick and tired, we often find ourselves contemplating where we lost control over our self-discipline as it concerns our healthy habits. Alternatively, we may play the blame game and think about what has been done to us through environmental factors, nutrition depletion in our food supply, or the abuse we have taken on our bodies from sitting all day long in our work chair. We might even resort to blaming our genes.

If you blame yourself and it motivates you to make better choices, that's fine. But you don't want to force yourself into a spiral of debilitation in the blame game. Beating yourself up for past mistakes in diet, exercise, and discipline won't do anything to build you back up to be the best version of yourself. That person who made choices yesterday is not the same person with the knowledge from this book.

Focusing on the things you cannot control (like the past) will only create more stress in your life, which will further deteriorate your health and well-being. So, if you are thinking about past mistakes, you are thinking of the wrong things! Let's look to a better future instead of being someone who is always busy looking back and questioning the past. You cannot live in the past *and* build a future at the same time. Let's focus our attention on where we are going, not where we have already been.

There are often many markers or signs when we're sick or *approaching* being sick. For that reason, it's critical to pay attention to what our bodies are telling us and act immediately. It is important to stay focused on diagnosing what is happening to you and within you, so that you can create a unique solution to your needs. The answers are available, but we need to start at the beginning and stop beating ourselves and others up. Let's save that energy for solutions, which will get us closer to our dream body, amazing health, and ultimate vitality!

In this section, I share some of the common issue areas where I find people are struggling and which lead to poor outcomes in their overall health. I suggest you look at each area so you can learn more about how your body works and what gets in the way of health and vitality. The more knowledgeable you are, the more you can help yourself and others reach a healthier existence.

OK, it's time to get down and dirty and learn the details of the human body. Let's dive in …

Endocrine System

The endocrine system is an incredibly powerful system that activates the rest of the body. It encompasses the hypothalamus, pituitary, thyroid, adrenal, and gonadal glands, to mention just a few of its primary components. Therefore, giving our hormones and neurotransmitters both dietary and lifestyle support is a primary concern in controlling homeostasis (balance) throughout our bodies and endocrine systems.

Sadly, many endocrine-related issues do not present until after prolonged damage has been done. A great example can be seen in many mid-life issues you might be familiar with. Sadly, in today's society, these issues are presenting earlier than ever before (including in teen years). Symptoms present in multiple ways, including:

- Hot flashes
- Hair loss
- Anxiety
- Belly fat

- Thyroid symptoms
- Adrenal fatigue
- Low testosterone
- Elevated estrogens

These symptoms, known as the "diseased state" in life, used to occur around the seventh or eighth decade of life. But each decade (starting around the '70s or '80s) they have started to present earlier and earlier in my patients. It is so troubling to see patients walk into the office in their teenage years with so many of these "used to be rare or nonexistent" symptoms.

Do any of these symptoms above describe you or someone you know?

Your Adrenals and That Pesky Adrenal Fatigue

Adrenal fatigue is far too common in my patients these days. As the world has increased in stressors (inflammatory diets, wars, stressed out/burnt out society, COVID-19, inflation), your adrenals have responded. Yet, the kind of stress we experience today is not the same as years ago, when stress was seemingly more fleeting. Today, people feel chronically stressed without any relief—especially caretakers.

Your adrenals respond to every kind of stress, no matter the source (period). Therefore, whenever possible, it is important to try to avoid stress triggers that induce an adrenal response. I know. I know. You are thinking "duh." Of course, we all know that we need to reduce stress and that it is bad for us, but I am telling you to *seriously* commit to finding ways to reduce stress—or else! "Or else, what?" you ask? Or else your body will go into a distressed mode, which leads to adrenal fatigue and a slew of symptoms that will eventually put you at risk for premature aging and even premature death!

So, how do you know if you are experiencing adrenal fatigue? And what causes it?

Chronic adrenal fatigue can become very complex, and the symptoms go on and on. Typical symptoms can include:

- Difficulty getting up in the morning
- Continuing fatigue not relieved by rest
- Cravings for salt or salty foods
- Lack of energy
- Lightheadedness when quickly standing up
- Mild depression
- Increased effort required to do everyday tasks
- Decreased sex drive
- Decreased ability to handle stress
- Increased time needed to recover from illnesses (COVID/flu), trauma, or injury
- Decreased enjoyment, lack of zest, or happiness with your life
- Increased PMS symptoms
- Symptoms increase when meals are skipped
- Thoughts are less focused, fuzzier
- Memory is less accurate
- Decreased tolerance
- Decreased productivity

Adrenal fatigue syndrome is regulated by the hypothalamus, the pituitary, and the adrenal gland pathway, known as the HPA Axis, and the number one cause is stress. Sound like anybody you know? It sounds like everybody I know!

Yes, the single greatest contributor to adrenal fatigue, or adrenal burnout, is stress. Stress can come at you in many forms, including via emotional, physical, conscious, and subconscious factors. Stress directly affects nearly everyone. It does not distinguish between race, social status, education, or blood type. The ultimate question isn't so much a matter of who *is* stressed—it's a matter of finding anyone who *isn't* stressed.

When looking for solutions to stresses in life, I always think of relationships first. They are key to good health and play a huge role in longevity. In the book *The Good Life* by Robert Waldinger, MD, and Marc Schulz, PhD, which shares information based upon a scientific study of happiness, they propose the key to dealing with stress is relationships. Our relationships are what keep us healthy and help us get past our everyday burdens. Seriously, think about it: It's not easy to get a good laugh on your own!

One key in relationships is laughter, which can lift us up even when we don't want to be lifted. It is hard to stay in a bad mood when you're laughing or even *hearing* others laugh. Yes, a key to health and longevity includes more laughter! Laughter can have a calming effect on our stress levels. Stress can:

- Promote inflammation
- Increase anxiety and depression
- Suppress immunity
- Encourage cancer growth
- Elevate blood pressure (which in turn raises the risk for strokes and heart attacks)
- Promote vascular disease
- Lead to insulin resistance
- Induce diabetes and obesity
- Impair cognitive and emotional circuits in the brain
- Elevate cortisol

How does stress do all this in your body, you ask?

Stress elevates the hormone **cortisol**. Cortisol elevation is common in individuals with blood sugar imbalances, which is commonly found in those with obesity, type II Diabetes, and cardiovascular disease—all of which are known to decrease life spans. It does not stop there. Cortisol elevation throws fuel on proinflammatory diseases like IBS, Crohn's, lupus, multiple sclerosis, rheumatoid arthritis, Sjogren's, all dermatitis syndromes, and more.

Cortisol imbalance is one of the **primary** causes of pre-mature aging and death. All inflammation throughout the body has a direct relationship with cortisol. I know that's scary, but don't' let it stress you out! There are answers for stressors in your life, which we will get to later in the book.

Stress often seems like it's everywhere—so, how can you get rid of it? Well, as with everything, balance and management are key. It is not about "getting rid" of it as much as it is transforming yourself to manage it better. There are so many ways to reduce stress, including taking more control over your health and nutrition.

The key is to develop a plan that works for you, work at it consistently, and reassess regularly when needed. What are things that you do to de-stress? What are things that have been successful in lessening your stress burden that you don't do anymore? For instance, did you know that taking a walk outside and getting some sunlight will help you reduce your stress? And yet, you don't make the effort anymore ... because you feel too stressed? Write down anything you can think of to help alleviate your stress. Then, talk to friends and family about how they cope with stress and ideas they have for you to reduce it. Develop a plan, because if you don't, your stressors will surely compound.

Yes, stress is here to stay, but there are ways to reduce it and redirect it in your life. For me, faith is a major support system in reducing my stress. I also make sure I do things that I enjoy, including working out regularly to keep my body functioning properly and taking time with my loved ones each day. I also take time for myself, even as a parent of a young toddler. When I get off track due to life circumstances, I develop a plan and stick to it. Planning saved my life. (See Part VI, What Can I Do? for more information on how you can develop a plan for life!)

"Trust in the Lord with all your heart and lean not on your own understanding; in all your ways submit to Him & He will make your plans straight."
Proverbs 3:5-6 (NIV)

Autonomic Disorders and the Adrenal/ Cortisol Stress Connection

Autoimmunity basically amounts to the body's assault on its own immune system—the very system that it is designed to defend. Most autoimmune diseases are considered idiopathic in nature, which basically means "We don't have a clue" or "Of unknown origin." So, if a cause cannot be identified, how do you go about developing a cure or reversal of a disease? These disorders are largely considered untreatable (endocrinologists included) due to the lack of adrenal fatigue syndrome education in the medical school's curriculum. The exception is full-blown adrenal exhaustion, which, if left untreated, could result in death.

According to Tabor's Encyclopedic Medical Dictionary, "Chronic maintenance of Addison's disease requires an increased dose of hormone replacement steroids during times of increased mental and physical stress. Because stress may precipitate a crisis, discuss stress management with the patient." That is the standard medical treatment plan—yes, drugs and stress management—for the absolute worst-case scenario of adrenal exhaustion. So, let's dig deeper for both a cause and a treatment focused on a resolution.

I personally believe nearly 100% of autonomic disorders have a connection between mind and body. I don't believe they are idiopathic. After all, they have a connection to prolonged nutritional and lifestyle health issues (usually associated with sub-threshold inflammation) that are primarily diet induced and exacerbated by a deep-rooted stress response. Perhaps the most frustrating problem associated with autonomic disorders is the prolonged course between the onset of symptoms and a diagnosis, which can sometimes be years.

These disorders are very hard to pinpoint due to lack of specific health markers for detection of autoimmune disorders, such as blood tests, physical exams, or image studies (like an X-ray or MRI). This results in further frustration and increased stress, anxiety, and full-blown illness before any proactive treatment is taken. If you are one of the lucky few, chances slim as they are, your endocrinologist may give you a diagnosis of an "idiopathic hypothalamus disorder," which is most likely considered untreatable by your physician. Again, none of this is surprising given adrenal fatigue and the many complications that come with it.

Sadly, this area is no longer taught at an appropriate level in most medical curriculum. No insurance ICD-10 codes even exist to bill for the related treatment of adrenal fatigue. Therefore, no reimbursement is allowable for treatment providers, which means no treatment protocol exists, and ultimately no care plan. Sorry!

Stay strong—your treatment options will improve. The treatment protocols are out there, and we will get to them shortly. But first, let's dive into a little more information. Knowledge is power, so let's gain some more!

These tiny little adrenal glands that sit above the kidneys are powerful regulators in the autonomic nervous system. As I mentioned earlier, full blown adrenal failure can result in death. Therefore, the adrenals will steal energy to function from surrounding endocrine glands (such as the thyroid, gonads, ovaries, etc.).

You can survive without your ovaries, ladies. And human beings can live past a thyroidectomy. However, adrenal gland removal is something we *cannot survive.* Sadly, most treating physicians are left with very few treatment alternatives. They treat with biologics, which have debilitating side effects (or should I just say *effects,*), or with anti-depressant prescriptions, which do nothing to address the underlying cause and provide only symptomatic relief, at best.

Now, let's look at some very interesting connections between adrenal fatigue and autoimmune disorder involving diet and hormones. In 1985, wheat was changed for good to ward off the hunger famine in Ethiopia. To be more specific, wheat was altered from a four-foot Amber grain (as the song reflects) to a two-foot dwarf that could be harvested at twice the frequency. This new grain also contained four times the gluten content. Interestingly, during this same period autonomic disorders (such as multiple sclerosis, lupus, rheumatoid arthritis, irritable bowel syndrome, and skin related inflammatory disorders) skyrocketed!

In my practice, I notice that 70% or greater of autoimmune disease sufferers are women. Many of these diseases result in disability and even death. In fact, lupus is significantly more likely to strike women, as is multiple sclerosis. Even rheumatoid arthritis is three times greater in women than men. What is happening?

My hypothesis is that there must be a link with the proinflammatory hormone estrogen, which is linked to most female cancers and prostate cancer in elderly males, whose estrogen levels increase with age in line with prostate disorders. Then, when you add estrogen-mimicking foods like soy and inflammatory glutens to the mix, you're just adding fuel to the fire. The result is HPA axis dysregulation.

The HPA axis is the stress regulating feedback loop between the hypothalamus, pituitary, and adrenal glands. Could restoring optimal regulation to this feedback loop system be the holy grail for re-booting and restoring adrenal function and ultimately getting a hold on this autonomic disorder? My clinical experiences have been wonderfully promising! Unfortunately, there is no protocol for treating the causes of stress or its ramifications like chronic fatigue syndrome, autonomic disorders, depression, or anxiety in our healthcare system outside of symptom suppressing medications.

The medical field will prescribe medications (sometimes multiple prescriptions) to ease their patients' symptoms—but that does not do anything to the underlying causes. In some cases, when there are unexplained symptoms and the tests all come back within the normal range of guidelines, patients are prescribed anti-depressants without a valid diagnosis to show for it. Doctors know that stress can be an underlying cause for most things, so this is not totally off base. That said, I fight to know and treat underlying causes before they get worse, including stress management, nutritional support, and supplementation.

Beyond the adrenals, stress is an enemy to numerous functions of your body!

Hypertension

Hypertension, also known as high blood pressure, is a long-term medical condition that can and often does go unnoticed. Some have called it a silent killer. Many have started accepting blood pressure issues as something "we all get" as we age. It does not have to be that way at all.

There is a reason your body increases its blood pressure. Your body is working to maintain a healthy supply of oxygen and nutrients to all the body's organs (including the brain). Keep in mind that everyone has a different ideal blood pressure. The medical community tries to make guidelines as if there is a one-size-fits-all answer, but those guidelines do not take unique characteristics into account.

Just as everyone has a different height and weight, they also have different blood sugar levels, cholesterol levels, etc. So, to say a male's blood pressure needs to be 120/80 and a female's blood pressure should be maintained at a reading level of 110/70 is ludicrous. For example, someone of a larger status and weight will have more blood capillaries that need to be filled and more oxygen to be transferred, thus requiring a greater blood pressure.

Just over 60 years ago, the first prescription blood pressure drugs appeared for lowering blood pressure. Back before these first prescription drugs were available, most physicians considered blood pressure markers to be one's age plus 100. That is:

- 20-year-olds: 120
- 40-year-olds: 140
- 60-year-olds: 160

Often it took much more than 180/95 in an 80-year-old to get much attention in what was known as the "100 plus the age" protocol. This method of measure is no longer used today in our over-regulated, over-medicated healthcare (sick care) system. We live in a society where the healthcare system is spending perhaps only one-tenth of its resources on preventing disease and nine-tenths of its resources on managing and profiting from sickness (it). Denying the fact that those profit motives exist is what is stopping any real progress in educating people on how to eat and live in a way to promote healthy lives.

Deny nothing and observe "what works." See clearly "what's so," and life becomes simple using these tools. Honor the process. Life, "the energy," is always there. It is never not there; life never ends.

Anti-hypertensive drugs are widely prescribed today. The logic seems simple: If high blood pressure is bad, lowering it must be good. People taking such medications will have fewer strokes and live longer, right? Research published in Joel Kauffman's *Malignant Medical Myths* shows this to be true only for people with very high blood pressure—those in the upper 10%. People are excited to take a magic pill, but few know that there are very significant side effects—so bad that over 50% of those prescribed stop taking them within three years (Kauffman, 105). The collateral damage can be so extreme for many people that no increase in lifespan is obtained. It is therefore not as easy of a decision to make as you might think.

How High is Considered Hypertension?

Blood pressure rises naturally with age, and it rises higher for females than males. Yet, females have a longer average life span. The "normal" levels most physicians tell males to strive to achieve is 120/80. Interestingly, this level is observed in only about 25% of adult males (Kauffman, 107). Most sources agreed back in the 1970s that normal resting blood pressure was 160/95 mg/hg for the average 50-year-old. Again, this is closer to the earlier guidelines of "age plus 100."

In order to favor the pharmaceutical industry, blood pressure values for this age group have dropped to 140/80 which is not patient optimal. Why such a drastic change in 30 years?

What Causes Hypertension?

Hypertension, in itself, is not a disease. It is a physical finding (a symptom) stemming from some other problem. This is a key component that I stress with my patients when they ask why their blood pressure is elevated. Simply popping a pill to regulate a number does absolutely nothing for treating the cause. Find *that* problem, address it, and remove the need for symptom regulation.

Blood pressure is unique to a person, and so is the cause. Simple everyday stress can increase blood pressure. Physical activity and emotional issues can cause a rise in blood pressure (though only temporarily). These can be considered healthy responses, as they bring additional oxygen for temporary physiological support. I even know people with a "white coat response." In this case, one's blood pressure elevates when they go to the doctor, only to decrease as they start to relax in the office.

What is known as *secondary hypertension* is what we really must identify and address. This causes either atherosclerosis of the arteries in the kidney (renal hypertension) or hepatic hypertension due to liver complications. Both organs are filter systems for our bodies, and addressing these issues (for example, via organ detoxification) will help restore blood pressure to normal. Also, a decrease in blood flow through these organs is compensated by an increase in blood pressure. Interfering with this natural process cannot possibly be of 100% benefit—again it is all about oxygen carrying and oxygen utilization.

The key here is that with hypertension, it is important to find the "why" if you wish to prevent a lifetime of medication and regulation of numbers (that some consider hypothetical). This is especially true when you consider the quality-of-life consequences from prolonged use. I say, let's get your overall health advancing in the right direction and you will see all those "numbers" get back on track and moving in the right direction. Again, I like to look at the underlying causes and the "whole" person.

Other endocrine disorders can also raise blood pressure. For example, consider stress, its effect on the adrenal glands, and elevation of inflammatory hormone cortisol. On top of that, there are the additional problems associated with stress, including diabetes, weight gain, and fluid retention. There is good news though ... almost every time, a 10-20-pound drop in weight results in decreased overall blood pressure. Read on to see how weight management can be your key to better health and vitality.

You can see results (like those of the claims you hear on TV for anti-hypertensive drugs) without bad side effects. When you identify and treat the underlying cause instead of just the symptoms, hypertension may be reduced with an overall benefit to the patient.

Keep in mind that the side effects of antihypertensive drugs go beyond just lowering blood pressure. These side effects can hit early in treatment, and more can come over long periods of time. As with any diagnosis and medication, you and your physician should be closely monitoring your progress. It is critical to monitor yourself in both early and lates stages of using a new prescription, as the impacts build up. Many reactions can be easily missed, especially when you are using various medications in tandem.

The body is always in a state of trying to maintain an adequate supply of oxygen and nutrients to its vital organs. And to achieve this, it keeps blood pressure only as high as necessary. Lowering one's blood pressure is, no surprise, always a stress to the body. Interfering with this natural process could cause trouble. An all too frequent example of this is the elderly using hypertension drugs with one of its main side effects being dizziness and hypotension (when blood pressure is too low). A serious low blood pressure issue is known as postural hypotension. An example of this is the all-too-common scenario of a person awakening in the middle of the night to use the bathroom, arising too quickly, and the sudden drop in blood pressure causes them to become dizzy. This results in a fall, increasing the possibility of a hip fracture or life-threatening head injury.

The cause of demise was not the head injury, but ultimately the low blood pressure. Here are a few key points to keep in mind when you are having your blood pressure checked. For starters, avoid stimulants like caffeine prior to testing. Also, consider stressors that might affect your resting blood pressure like traffic, relationship issues, white coat syndrome, or any other outside occurrences that could elevate your results.

In my opinion, drugs should only be prioritized as an option for those with extreme hypertension—perhaps the top 20% of the hypertensive population. Again, we must create a unique plan for *you*. In my practice, I am conservative when it comes to treatment of my patients. I know the body can do amazing things to cure itself.

My recommendation is to first focus on what is happening within your body—things *you* can control. I suggest moving to a low carbohydrate diet, magnesium supplementation (see the aspirin chapter in *Medical Myths*), fish oils, and natural vasodilators like L-arginine and testosterone therapy. Even if you only see partial success under that plan, diet and supplementation will allow you to use much lower doses of drugs. This means fewer side-effects.

Most importantly, if your hypertension is the result of what is termed "secondary hypertension" such as hepatic (liver) or renal (kidney), or blood sugars (as seen in type II diabetes), the best approach is to identify the cause and correct the problem so as not to create more health issues later. Primary hypertension from physical activity and emotional stress often corrects itself.

When it comes to your health, I say leave no stone unturned. The goal is to get you back to feeling great, energized, and full of life for the long haul! Do what it takes. The sky is the limit when we invest in ourselves and, more importantly, our health!

Fibromyalgia and Chronic Fatigue Syndrome

These two diseases, which are often described as epidemics today, are in most cases little more than vitamin and mineral deficiencies and the over-utilization of sugars or processed foods. Refined sugars and carbohydrates deplete the body's B-complex vitamin storage and are harder to metabolize and use for energy in the form of adenosine triphosphate (ATP). Think of ATP as the fuel that runs the body, much like gasoline runs your car. ATP is the product of what is called aerobic cellular respiration (A.K.A. the Krebs or citric acid cycle).

Our bodies require B-complex vitamins and other minerals to make the Krebs cycle function. But most American diets are lacking sufficient B-complex vitamins. Unfortunately, these nutrients are depleted in our diets, most specifically B1 (thiamine) and the minerals manganese, magnesium, and iodine. Again, it's pharmaceuticals (medications) and processed foods that are a major contributor for this depletion. Lack of these nutrients makes the absorption of pyruvic acid into the Krebs (energy) cycle difficult. This causes a buildup of lactic acid in our muscle and connective tissues, leading to chronic muscle soreness and pain. This is diagnosed as fibromyalgia, with side effects of chronic fatigue.

B-complex vitamins are found highest in raw liver, nutritional yeast, and the germ portion of uncooked brans and sprouted grains—all foods not commonly found in American diets. Thus, we need proper whole food supplements—not the mega-high dosages of synthetic B-vitamins produced by laboratories from Coal Tar, which only exacerbate an already existing B-complex deficiency.

Another major contributor of vitamin B deficiencies in American diets is consumption of fortified bread, which has shown to leach B vitamin reserves from our bodies. To comprehend the chronic fatigue syndrome caused by vitamin and mineral deficiency diets, look again at the conversion of glucose to ATP through the Krebs cycle.

Various nutrients are necessary to make the Krebs cycle function, including thiamine (B1), riboflavin (B2), niacinamide (B3), manganese, magnesium, iodine, and phosphorous, to name a few. One molecule of glucose completely utilized through the Krebs cycle yields 36 molecules of ATP energy. On the other hand, a single molecule of glucose not completely utilized through the Krebs cycle yields only six molecules of ATP.

So, it's no wonder we run out of energy so quickly. Think of this scenario as trying to heat your home fireplace using nothing but paper. It burns quickly, and then it's gone—and so is the heat (i.e., your energy).

Acid Reflux

Antacid is the wrong biochemistry because it neutralizes one of the most important of all body secretions: hydrochloric acid (HCL). This prevents the stomach from performing the sole purpose it was designed for—*producing* hydrochloric acid. The manufactures of pharmaceuticals like Nexium and Prevacid (i.e., protein pump inhibitors) want you to believe the cause of acid reflux and esophageal disease is an overly acidic stomach—but that is an oxymoron. The reality is the exact opposite. Instead, acid reflux occurs when the stomach becomes too alkaline.

The effects of acid reflux can be minor or severe and can interfere with daily activities. Acid reflux is a very common condition. In fact, most of us know people of all ages suffering from acid reflux, and the effects can be minor or severe and can interfere with daily activities. Thankfully, there are answers to acid reflux that don't create more health problems like the side effects associated with medications. These answers boil down to lifestyle changes.

A simple example of this is the use of apple cider vinegar before a meal, which has proven to help so many people avoid reflux symptoms. When they consume apple cider vinegar before a meal, digestion is improved due to your body's ability to increase acidity in the stomach, thus improving digestion.

Western diets today are void of the necessary enzymes our food should have. Why? Because everything is processed, which increases shelf life and prevents spoiling. Lack of these enzymes puts a heavy stress on our body's natural digestive and pancreatic enzymes. This often diminishes our nutritional reserves earlier and earlier from generation to generation—resulting in acid reflux and nutritional deficiency disorders at alarmingly younger ages.

When you add in medications, high-carbohydrate diets, and the consumption of dead calories like soft drinks and alcohol, it's no wonder the natural, optimal HCL levels in your stomach are depleting at such an alarming rate. This leaves us unable to break down stomach contents and nutrients (namely proteins and minerals) in a timely manner due to insufficient digestive enzymes like the protein enzyme pepsin.

Due to the slowed digestion rate of the proteins, the more simply digestive foods—like carbohydrates, and *especially* processed carbs— are broken down. This creates a gaseous secretion that causes bloating, gas pressure, and stomach expansion through the diaphragm. This often results in hiatal herniation and reflux problems.

Why does modern science and mankind think it's logical to stop our natural physiology by preventing normal stomach function of acid production and reversing it into an alkaline organ? It's beyond my comprehension. It is not the way we were designed to be, and it's just another example of man-made regulation through medication—not your definition of healthy. So, perhaps the cure for acid reflux lies in restoring proper HCl levels in the stomach, which will enable adequate function as it was designed by our Creator. It will also help us avoid side effects of inadequate stomach acid such as anemia, muscle cramping, restless legs, bone loss, and protein and mineral deficiencies.

Acid reflux, also known as gastroesophageal reflux disease (GERD), is a common condition that affects millions of people worldwide. It occurs when stomach acid and other digestive juices flow back up into the esophagus, the tube that connects the throat and the stomach. This can cause a burning sensation in the chest, commonly known as heartburn.

Symptoms of acid reflux can include heartburn, regurgitation of food or liquid, difficulty swallowing, coughing, and a sour or bitter taste in the mouth. These symptoms can be mild or severe and may occur on a regular basis, interfering with daily activities and reducing quality of life.

There are several factors that can contribute to the development of acid reflux, including:

1. **Poor eating habits.** Eating large meals, consuming spicy or acidic foods, and eating late at night can all contribute to acid reflux.
2. **Obesity.** Excess weight can put pressure on the stomach, causing acid reflux.
3. **Hiatal hernia.** This occurs when part of the stomach protrudes through the diaphragm and into the chest cavity, which can increase the likelihood of acid reflux. (See Hiatal Hernia Figure 4.1 for more information.)
4. **Pregnancy.** The hormone progesterone can relax the valve that separates the esophagus from the stomach, leading to acid reflux.
5. **Smoking.** Tobacco use can weaken the valve between the esophagus and the stomach, making acid reflux more likely.
6. **Medications.** Certain medications, including some antidepressants and blood pressure medications, can contribute to acid reflux.

Side effects of inadequate stomach acid include, but are not limited to:

- Anemia
- Muscle cramping
- Restless legs
- Bone loss
- Protein and minerals deficiencies

However, please note that most people will not be able to come off prolonged use of antacids or protein pump inhibitors (like Nexium) abruptly, as they may experience acid rebound issues. Instead, they will need to start an HCL and digestive enzyme protocol to establish proper stomach function before gradually reducing medication use. Visit www.DrJoeyJones.com to learn more about improving HCL reserves and restoring proper stomach function.

A hiatal hernia occurs when the upper part of your stomach bulges through your diaphragm (the large muscle separating your abdomen and chest) and into your chest cavity. Most small hiatal hernias cause no signs or symptoms. However, a larger hiatal hernia can cause heartburn, regurgitation of food or liquids into the mouth, acid reflux, difficulty swallowing, chest pain or abdominal pain, feeling full soon after you eat, and shortness of breath. Hiatal hernias are caused by an increase in carb-forming gas due to a lack of enzymes, which are no longer commonly found in many foods. A key missing component, for example, is pepsin for protein.

I offer non-invasive treatment options for hiatal hernias that includes gentle, manual therapy to reduce the hernia and eventually eliminate it. I also recommend hydrochloric acid (HCL) and enzyme supplementation to restore normal stomach function. My treatment plan focuses on treating the primary cause of hiatal hernias, which eliminates the need for symptom suppression. Visit www.DrJoeyJones. com to learn more about my gentle, non-invasive approach.

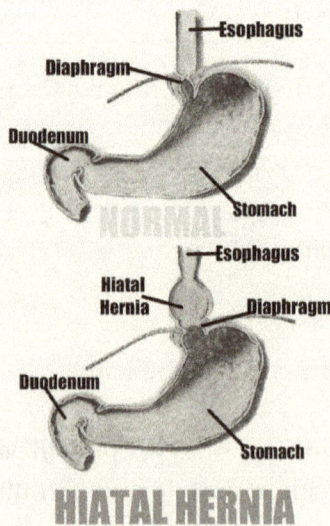

Figure 4.1

Cholesterol

Cholesterol does the body good and is an absolute essential ingredient to good health. For example, without cholesterol, the body would be incapable of producing life-sustaining steroid hormones. Growing bodies of research suggest that drugs and even diets that drastically reduce cholesterol levels in the body may be doing more harm than good. This is partly because they limit the precursor materials that steroids can produce.

In my opinion, the harmful side effects of using statin drugs to reduce serum cholesterol levels may far outweigh the benefits. Considering my research over the last 20+ years, I find drug treatments reduce one's quality of life and possibly their overall life span almost as much and as fast as hyperinsulinemia (type II diabetes). Nothing, and I repeat, *nothing*, will decline your overall health faster than a statin drug. (Well ... maybe a protein pump inhibitor, such as antacids for controlling acid reflux.)

No assertions are made here without evidence. I have read this in top-selling books over the past few years, such as:

- *The Magic of Cholesterol Numbers* by Sergey A. Dzugan, MD, PHD
- *The Great Cholesterol Con* by Dr. Malcolm Kendrick
- *The Great Cholesterol Con* by Anthony Colpo

These books are a must-read for everyone, including physicians and all "would be" statin drug patients. "New research reveals statin drugs may lessen brain function and increase risk for heart disease" says Joel M. Kauffman, Ph.D., in *Malignant Medical Myths* (Kauffman, 78-101).

When taking statins, you might think, "Wait, doctor, what am I taking this drug for?" In fact, before you know it, you may be on a long list of drugs for one symptom that only leads you to taking more drugs for symptoms caused by the original drug. In *Grain Brain*, Dr. David Perlmutter, M.D., writes, "The alleged correlation between high cholesterol and high cardiac risk is an absolute fallacy. The public is being deceived by the greatest health scam of the century."

Death by Statins

Is It Slow Suicide? You Decide.

Statin drug toxicity is a consequence of CoQ10 depletion and cellular disfunction. The body must have adequate hormone production, testosterone, and estrogen to break down protein waste byproducts. These processes include eliminating toxins out of connective tissues via the mitochondria to prevent protein debris, waste product buildup, and subsequent acidic byproducts that cause cellular destruction and death, thus preventing cellular mitosis and regeneration. Statin drugs destroy CoQ10, thus decreasing mitochondria growth and inhibiting the removal of toxic waste.

A lack of CoQ10 also leads to the absence of hormone production, which is caused by the blockage of the HMG-CoA reductase pathway (which is responsible for cholesterol synthesis, a necessary precursor to hormone production). If you eliminate CoQ10, life cannot exist because mitochondria cannot produce energy. Yet statin drugs do just that, halting the synthesis of both cholesterol and CoQ10.

This also disrupts a toxic elimination pathway, which results in toxic waste and debris buildup in the tissue and leads to nerve and muscle toxicity conditions such as myopathy and neuropathy. Next comes further cellular destruction, telomere damage, an increased rate of cellular aging, and an increased rate of cellular death. In other words: It's a form of suicide by slowly suffocating cells over time.

Let me be clear—I am not telling you to personally stop taking your statin medication. I'm telling you that if I were responsible for your health care, I would 100% choose an alternative, less toxic approach.

I would recommend anyone taking statin medications to monitor their CoQ10 levels and supplement 200-600 mg of Coenzyme Q10 daily.

To learn more about statin side effects and alternative recommendations, visit www.DrJoeyJones.com.

Physiology 101 shows that carbohydrates stimulate insulin, which in turn triggers fatty acid synthesis in the liver. This in turn floods the bloodstream with triglycerides, the real bad guys. Again, it's carbohydrate consumption from foods like enriched wheat flour that increases total cholesterol, LDLs, and triglycerides.

Fat and protein have little to no effect on triglycerides or total cholesterol. In fact, both are elevated by carbohydrates. Let's dive into the facts:

Fact: It is low-fat, "healthy whole grain" (i.e., carbohydrate-rich) diets that increase cholesterol and triglycerides.

- To quote the world-renowned cardiologist and #1 bestselling author of *Wheat Belly*, William Davis, MD: "If carbohydrates, such as wheat, trigger the entire domino effect of VLDL/triglyceride/small LDL particles, then reducing carbohydrates should do the opposite, particularly the dominating carbohydrate wheat."

Fact: Statin drugs work their cardiovascular effect not by manipulating cholesterol, but simply by their now well-established anti-inflammatory role.

- It's true—doctors can reduce cardiovascular risk with statins, though only very slightly. This is done primarily through statins' role as an anti-inflammatory.
- Side effects to overall physiological disruption in the body are frightening to say the least—especially when one considers the same benefits of natural anti-inflammatory alternatives such as fish oils, flaxseed, turmeric, vitamin C, vitamin B, buckwheat, magnesium, etc.
- Statin drugs lower serum cholesterol by inhibiting the production of other vital intermediary metabolic pathways necessary for longevity and vitality, such as coenzyme Q10, DHEA, and sex hormones like testosterone and estrogen.
- In *Malignant Medical Myths*, Joel M. Kauffman writes, "Doing so by stopping biosynthesis of cholesterol in the liver

by using drugs will be shown to be undesirable, since there is so much collateral damage."

Serum total cholesterol rises naturally with age:

- Mean level of 178mg/dL in 18–24-year-olds rises to a maximum level of around 230 mg/dL in 55–60-year-olds
  - Men and women over the age of 55 who have high cholesterol levels typically live longer than those with cholesterol levels *below* 200
  - High total cholesterol protects against cardiovascular disease and CVD infections. Yes, you read that right! If needed, read it again and let it sink in!

- As we age, most hormones (like sex hormones) tend to decline. This trend is known throughout science and endocrinology.

Cholesterol is a powerful precursor for all hormone production, thus elevated cholesterol may often be the body's attempt to upregulate declining hormone output.

METABOLISM OF CHOLESTEROL
(SIMPLIFIED VERSION)

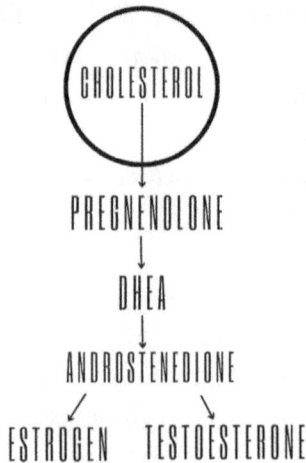

CHOLESTEROL

PREGNENOLONE

DHEA

ANDROSTENEDIONE

ESTROGEN   TESTOESTERONE

Figure 4.2

When the average middle-aged patient visits their doctor and has their blood drawn, seldom, if ever, is any attention given to the patient's hormone levels (except perhaps vitamin D). This is probably because few doctors truly understand hormones and shy away from testing what they don't comprehend.

So, your lipid panels get tested, and your cholesterol comes back "elevated" above 200. This "elevated" number, by the way, was chosen by pharmaceutical companies to maximize their return on investments for scam research and development reimbursement. It's no surprise that ¼ of the American population had cholesterol levels over this number, meaning pharmaceutical companies could immediately profit off their health issues. This is *SCARY!*

Back to our patient. With no regard for the patient's hormonal dysfunction, he or she is prescribed a statin drug to lower total cholesterol under the hypothetical scam that it will reduce cardiac risk. Many physicians fail to consider the bigger picture and the physiological response to hormonal imbalances associated with inadequate cholesterol levels.

Females will suffer many of the same effects from hormonal imbalances. And men with low "T" levels tend to have the following heart-related issues, which are signs of hormonal imbalances that tend to be overlooked in favor of statin drug prescriptions:

- High blood cholesterol
- High blood triglycerides
- Atherosclerosis
- Diabetes
- High blood glucose
- High blood pressure
- High body mass index (obesity)
- Angina pectoris (chest pain)
- High levels of blood clotting factors
- Low levels of blood clotting inhibitors.

*Side note: Pay attention to how many of the side effects will be treated by another pharmaceutical drug.

Are you still not sold on the fact that there is mainstream misinformation and misrepresentation on cholesterol? Here's another quote based off scientific studies in *Malignant Medical Myths,* "Even screening for cholesterol is not worthwhile and is said to be a waste of resources of the UK's National Health Services, since it is such a poor predictor of who will have cardiovascular disease."

In my opinion, there has never been satisfactory evidence that lowering total cholesterol or LDLs in most people is of any benefit. While correlation does not necessarily prove a cause, a lack of correlation does prove lack of cause.

Again, there is no evidence for improvement of well-being when taking a statin drug! My experience with patients has been quite the opposite, actually. If use of such a drug continues long enough, side effects tend to include:

- Congestive heart failure, dementia, amnesia, liver damage, kidney damage, muscle damage, nerve damage, respiratory problems, cognitive deficit, a possible 50% increase in diagnosis of Alzheimer's disease, loss of libido, erectile dysfunction, cancer, chronic fatigue, irritability, swelling in the legs, and much more

I mean ... come on! Like we don't already have enough challenges as we attempt to navigate the current issues affecting our long-term health.

Someone, anyone, please show me one case where the actual cause of someone's death was labeled high cholesterol. Just one. I'm not asking for two, just one. In my practice of 30+ years, I have seen countless cases of chronic sciatica, myopathy, and neuropathy cases resolve themselves when patients discontinue statin drug use.

Insulin

What one major component do all the longest living individuals and organisms have in common? I'll tell you: low insulin levels, which are perhaps the single greatest marker for a longer life. This is true be it yeast cells, insects, or mammals, including human beings. How much insulin we produce over the course of our lifetime plays a major role in how long we live. So, the less insulin we produce and subsequently need, the better it is for longevity.

Insulin blood tests measure the amount of the hormone insulin in the blood that is produced and stored in beta cells in our pancreas. Insulin helps regulate blood glucose levels and has a role in lipid (fat) metabolism.

When your body's response to insulin secretion is impaired (i.e., insulin resistance) (see Figure 4.3), your cells resist insulin's effects. This results in unhealthy, high blood glucose levels and metabolic related disorders like obesity, type II diabetes, neurological issues, and vision problems. Early symptoms usually present the following issues with low blood glucose (hypoglycemia):

- Sweating
- Palpitations
- Anxiety
- Dizziness
- Blurred vision
- Fainting
- Confusion
- Serious conditions like seizures and loss of consciousness

Insulin issues should also be considered in polycystic ovarian syndrome (PCOS), sleep apnea, abnormal skin conditions, and metabolic syndrome.

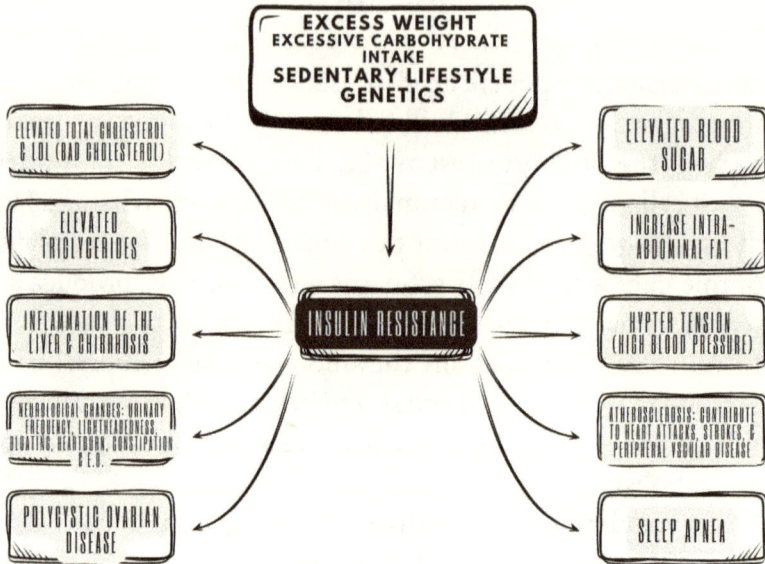

Figure 4.3

Medical Myth:
Aspirin for Preventing Heart Attacks

What you haven't heard about the debate of "one aspirin a day for primary prevention of heart attacks," and what I'm sure aspirin companies don't want you to know, is that the primary study [PHS 89] used *buffered* aspirin—aspirin mixed with magnesium (Kauffman, 17). And numerous studies have proven magnesium's powerful, protective effects on the heart. It dilates blood vessels, aids potassium distribution into cells (preventing heartbeat irregularities like arrythmias), acts as a natural blood thinner, and keeps blood cells from clumping together (i.e., an anti-platelet effect).

The study goes on to state that there was no difference in the death rate between aspirin vs. magnesium groups. However, the aspirin group had a 47% higher rate of deaths from *other* causes. To again quote Kauffman, "Stop taking that daily aspirin—stick to magnesium instead." Note, there is also no risk of peptic ulcers or hemorrhagic complications with magnesium use.

To sum up Kauffman's research, "Magnesium, vitamin E, certain omega-3 fatty acids, and the coenzyme Q10 provide much greater long-term benefits than aspirin—all with no negative side effects." The key component to be taken from the research in *Malignant Medical Myths* is that that none of the scientists had a dog in the hunt. They had no financial interest from pharmaceuticals or other outside interest.

Riddle me this: When someone is rushed to the emergency room for a cardiac event or stroke, what are they hooked up on? An aspirin or Bufferin drip? No, they're put on magnesium for its vasodilation, anti-coagulation, muscle relaxation, and natural blood thinning capabilities. That alone speaks volumes about the debate of magnesium over aspirin.

Testosterone Myths

Myth: Testosterone supplementation increases prostate cancer growth.

Fact (from the book *Testosterone for Life*, by Abraham Morgentaler, M.D., a must read for all men and physicians wanting the latest facts in testosterone health):

- "Raising T levels beyond the normal range did not seem to increase cancer growth even in men with metastatic cancer disease" (Morgentaler, 129).
- "For over 65 years, there has been a fear that T therapy will cause new prostate cancers to rise and hidden ones to grow. It is quite remarkable to discover that the long-standing fear about testosterone and prostate cancer has little scientific support" (Morgentaler, 135-136).

*Based on published evidence at the time of this book's writing:

- **Low** blood levels of testosterone may **increase** the risk of prostate cancer

- **High** blood levels of testosterone **do not** increase the risk of prostate cancer
- Treatment with testosterone **does not** increase risk of prostate cancer even among men at high risk for it (Morgentaler, 135)

For men who do have metastatic prostate cancer and who have been given treatment that drops their blood levels of testosterone to near zero (castration levels), starting treatment with testosterone might increase the risk that residual cancer will start to grow (Morgentaler, 136).

The Challenge Today

It is becoming more difficult to treat patient in today's healthcare (sick care) system, where the treatment protocol is designed around the ICD 10 insurance code and the diagnoses assigned to it. An **example** would be → Diagnosis: _____ → Gets prescription X, Y, and Z →.

Doctors must follow this protocol or be held liable for practicing outside of the recommended guidelines for the proposed "best way" to treat a diagnosis. So, there is more to your health care than your health and your doctor. You need to research and go to the doctor with questions—lots of questions!

Hang in there ... good news is coming later in the book!

Your Reflection Corner

Chapter 4: What Has Happened and Is Happening to Me?

Be in the know.

According to a study published in the Journal of the American Medical Association (JAMA), over 100,000 people die each year in the United States due to adverse drug reactions to properly prescribed medications. This number is based on data from 1994, so one can only imagine what the opioid crisis has done to that already staggering number. Regardless of what the number might be now, that's far too many deaths!

My point is that there is a reason for some medications to be taken. Just make sure it is your best option and that you have carefully assessed your health needs.

Take a few moments and listen to your body. Think about what is and is not working as it should be. Ask yourself *why* it's not working. Think about what the doctors have told you. Think about the information in this book. Now, write down the medications that you are taking and really think about what they are doing to your health and your body. Then ask yourself:

- Is it time to revisit them with your doctor?
- Is it time to research the medications you're on and your initial diagnosis?
- Is it time to retest and reexamine your approach to wellness?
- It is time to look at alternative approaches—like lifestyle and nutritional changes—that you can make?
- Is it time to take action?

After you have taken an inventory, if you have an urgent matter that needs to be addressed, call your doctor or pharmacist as soon as possible!

And if you want to dive deeper into some of the topics in this book, please visit my website at www.DrJoeyJones.com for continually refreshed information regarding your body, health, and longevity.

Do You Know?

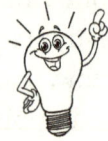

Varicose and Spider Veins

Tip: Rule out venous congestion issues and a possible liver connection.

Clue: Hemorrhoids. When looking for a possible underlying cause, consider what is called "loss of vascular integrity, capillary fragility, or vascular tone." The key is to repair and prevent these burst, inflamed, ruptured capillaries using what are known as anti-fragility factors found in the vitamin C complex. FYI: These c-complex factors are not found in most vitamin C products, such as ascorbic acid supplements. Again, a culprit to vascular issues can be venous congestion, as seen with liver congestion issues, which often respond well to liver detox and decongestion protocols.

CHAPTER 5

HOW DID THIS HAPPEN?

WITHIN ONE GENERATION OF THE food commerce takeover, our food supply became bleached, refined, chemically preserved, pasteurized, sterilized, homogenized, hydrogenated, artificially colored, defibered, highly sugared, highly salted, synthetically fortified ("enriched"), canned, and generally exposed to hundreds of new man-made chemicals. SORRY, WELCOME TO YOUR WORLD!

As we age, we must be deliberate in caring for our bodies if we wish to have the same health we had yesterday! And as you live longer, you may become more susceptible to illness and disease, so an effort must be made now to reverse that trend. In other words, if you focus on prevention, you will be less likely to suffer a diagnosis and treatment.

There have been increased trends in certain diseases and health outcomes due to our changes in lifestyle and diet over the years. For instance, the more sedentary lifestyle of many, because of COVID-19, has led to increased obesity, which creates greater risk of diabetes and other obesity-related illnesses. The older you get, the more diligent you must be with your diet and overall health. When we take care of our body, it will take care of us!

Being diligent about our health can have numerous positive impacts on our lives, including:

- Better overall quality of life – Nothing is more valuable than your health. Life is better experienced with good health, including having the energy to enjoy all that you have built over a lifetime of independence. The better you feel, the longer you can work to create the retirement you seek and have earned.

- Reduced health care costs – Do you want your hard-earned retirement dollars spent on family, bucket lists, boats, cars, indulgences, and vacations? Or do you want to give those dollars away to the healthcare system with little reward?
- Longevity – Don't you want to stick around for those grandchildren or to write that novel you always intended to write?
- Increased productivity – The better you feel, the more fulfillment you can have in your life, making everything you do even better.
- Setting a good example – If you live a wellness lifestyle, you can affect all around you for generations to come.

Look, it's time to get real about your health! Here are some staggering statistics to get you motivated:

According to the Center for Disease Control and Prevention (CDC) (https://www.cdc.gov/), as of 2019, 13% of the US adult population has diabetes.

According to the CDC, a large amount of the 2.8 million deaths in the U.S. were preventable.

In 2020, according to the American Heart Association (https://www.heart.org/), 655,000 died from heart disease.

According to the American Cancer Society (https://www.cancer.org/), in 2020, 1.6 million new cases of cancer were diagnosed in the US.

Society Health Issues

Most societal related health problems are not public health problems at all. They are not epidemics in the epidemiological sense. They are just the result of millions upon millions of individually responsible decisions—day in and day out. A large portion of our health outcomes are a result of our lifestyle choices, including self-imposed afflictions. Yes, there are diseases, but many of them are preventable or could have different outcomes with better choices.

These diseases are also exacerbated by social, political, economic, and environmental conditions. However, you have more ability to take control of your health and your outcomes than you know. With knowledge comes power. Power then brings control, and control instills confidence to establish your own path to radiant health.

Awareness is key. When trying to achieve optimal well-being, societal issues cannot be ignored. There are direct connections like having access to clean water, nutritious food, and safe housing. Yet there are other indirect impacts lurking around, too—like violence, which can stand in the way of well-being and your ability to experience a radiant life. Your stress levels directly impact your body. And by reducing social stressors alone, you can experience tremendous benefits.

Even so, no matter what societal impacts you face, you have more power than you know. In a later chapter, we will talk about how changing your mindset can change your health outcomes for the better—even if you don't do anything else.

Chronic Stress and Anxiety

Stress Kills

Stress increases cortisol levels and c-reactive protein levels, both of which are major precursors to a shortened life span. Stress related behaviors (including behaviors such as smoking, drinking, and overeating) will also decrease your life expectancy. These behaviors and stress alone will increase hypertension, as we talked about earlier.

I know there are a lot of valid reasons for you to feel stressed, but trust me, you cannot afford it! Yes, a stressed budget due to the costs of health care may make life more stressful—but that is *exactly* why you need to turn the tide on your health. The cost of health care, housing, and education are consuming ever larger shares of household budgets and rising faster than our incomes. You may not be able to control the housing market or skyrocketing food costs and education fees, but your health is yours to control, so own it!

The key to keeping rising health care costs down is to *not need* health care in the first place! You cannot trust Medicare or the government to care for you later in life when your income is fixed, and your health care costs consume the bulk of your savings. So, start by spending your current resources (both your time and expenses) on education about prevention of disease. And start to supplement nutritional support when your diet is inadequate.

Controlling Chronic Stress and Anxiety

Chronic stress/anxiety can bring down the strongest of individuals. Two tiny glands sitting atop your kidneys (called the adrenal glands) are responsible for handling our body's stress response. Stress and anxiety place a heavy burden on your nervous system and wreak havoc on your adrenal glands. Stress also over-stimulates your pancreas, causing extreme fluctuations in blood sugar and disrupting your sleep rhythms. How do you rank in your stress response? Do you have any of the issues below?

- Difficulty falling asleep
- Falling asleep, but then waking up and not being able to go back to sleep
- Waking up tired in the morning
- Mid-section obesity, which is difficult to lose

These are all signs of dysfunctional or stressed adrenal glands. Stress can be one of the toughest conditions to treat due to the multiple conditions that can cause it. And until the true underlying cause of one's stress is identified and addressed (i.e., job, marriage, health, family, etc.), the condition will continue to haunt you. It can take time to uncover the true underlying cause of the things stressing you. Some people don't wish to confront the cause, fearing it will bring even greater stress and anxiety. To see additional signs of adrenal fatigue, go to www.DrJoeyJones.com.

Unfortunately, there is no protocol for treating the causes of stress or its ramifications (like chronic fatigue syndrome, autonomic disorders, depression, or anxiety) in our healthcare system today. The typical medical response to a patient with chronic stress and anxiety includes prescribing medications that will only ease their symptoms. To me, this is a pity and unfair to the patient, who needs a more holistic view of their health.

There are answers out there, though. I lay out my action plan for stress management in a later chapter focused on solutions for your health.

Caregivers – Their Amazing Roles in Our Stressed-out Society

The number of caregivers in our society today is increasing at alarming rates. Caregivers for catastrophic injuries and disabilities such as autism, Alzheimer's, Parkinson's, and ALS are increasing year after year. The toll on these caregivers' stress regulators (mind, body, and spirit) is beyond my comprehension. Sadly, the magnitude in cost both financially and spiritually to those responsible for the lives of these precious souls is still not receiving its desired recognition at the healthcare and societal levels.

One can only imagine the stresses associated with caring for another's safety and well-being 24 hours a day, 365 days a year. Not having holiday relief, seldom getting deep REM sleep, and not getting enough breaks like going out to dinner can weigh heavily on the subconscious mind. Your fight, flight, or freeze mechanism is on 24/7 as a caregiver. It's like being a lifeguard all day, every day.

During challenging times, your mindset is key to keeping you out of bed and charging forward. Stress will burden all of us at one time or another, but caregivers experience all sorts of stress continuously. If you want to read an inspirational book about a caregiver's journey, I suggest you read Kimberly Kelsoe Hawkins's *Lessons Learned ... Through No Words at All*. Kimberly's book made me better understand the daily pressures of caretaking and how she rises above those pressures. Even if you aren't a caregiver now, this book is a good read on keeping a positive mindset despite *whatever* challenges you face. In her book, Kimberly shares the lessons she has learned through navigating life with twins—one of whom is diagnosed with multiple disabilities, including autism and being non-verbal.

The sympathetic nervous system that controls our fight or flight response—usually designed to get us out of life-threatening situations—is currently overloaded. There is seldom any time for resting, but it is never combined with the same relaxation others may get during restful periods. Special quality support is needed for schooling and activities. In addition, there is a very heavy burden beyond both physical and mental exhaustion, as the financial burdens keep soaring.

Clinical testing findings show that nearly all inflammatory markings are elevated in special caregivers, including:

- Elevated cortisol markers
- Elevated C-reactive protein
- Elevated homocysteine
- Increased anti-depressant use
- Poor metabolic function
- Abnormal distribution of fat
- Shortened telomere lengths (more on telomeres in a moment)

Yes, caregiving can be very rewarding, but it can also take a heavy toll on the caregiver, especially if they are going it alone. One can only imagine the stress on these caregivers' adrenal glands and their need for HPA axis regulation and support.

One study shared in the Journal of Gerontological Nursing found that caregivers report high stress levels (including depression and anxiety) when caring for individuals diagnosed with dementia. This study also reported that caregivers with these increased stress levels were more likely to report physical health problems.[2] Another study, this time from the Journal of Applied Social Psychology, reported higher levels of stress and lower well-being for caregivers

---

[2] Chiu, Y. C., Huang, H. L., & Liang, J. (2019). The relationship between stress and physical health among dementia caregivers: The moderating role of social support. Journal of Gerontological Nursing, 45(4), 35-41

of individuals diagnosed with Alzheimer's disease than the control group. They referred to the stress level as being comparable to that reported by military personnel during deployment.[3]

HPA Axis

If you are looking at management of stress and the body, look no further than the HPA axis (also known as the hypothalamic-pituitary-adrenal system). The HPA axis plays a key role in the regulation of stress. It's also the stress regulating feedback loop between the hypothalamus, pituitary, and adrenal glands.

The hypothalamus is the hub of the body and brain's stress apparatus, a key modulator of immune activity and the apex of the autonomic (limbic) nervous system. It is the transducer—our mind's eye into physiological data relating to our emotional behavioral, arousal, memory, and meaningful experiences. It translates fear, loss, grief, and stress into responses in our blood stream, organs, cells, nerves, lymph nodes, messenger chemicals, and molecules throughout the entire organism.

The hypothalamus is a small area of the brain located just above the brainstem. It plays a crucial role in regulating many bodily functions, including body temperature, hunger, thirst, and sleep. It also plays a significant role in our stress responses by releasing a hormone called corticotropin-releasing hormone (CRH) in response to stress.

Once released, CRH travels to the pituitary gland, which is a small gland located at the base of the brain. The pituitary gland produces and releases the adrenocorticotropic hormone (ACTH) in response to CRH. ACTH then travels to the adrenal glands on top of the kidneys.

The adrenal glands release cortisol, which is a steroid hormone that helps the body respond to stress. Cortisol has many effects on

---

[3] Mausbach, B. T., Aschbacher, K., Patterson, T. L., von Känel, R., Dimsdale, J. E., Mills, P. J., ... & Grant, I. (2007). Effects of placement and bereavement on psychological well-being and cardiovascular risk in Alzheimer's caregivers: A longitudinal analysis. Journal of Applied Social Psychology, 37(8), 1875-1903.

the body, including increasing blood sugar levels, suppressing the immune system, and increasing blood pressure. It also helps the body respond to stress by providing energy and increasing alertness.

The HPA axis is tightly regulated by a feedback system to maintain balance in the body. When cortisol levels are too high, the hypothalamus and pituitary gland will decrease their release of CRH and ACTH, which in turn will reduce cortisol levels. When cortisol levels are too low, the hypothalamus and pituitary gland will increase their release of CRH and ACTH, which will increase cortisol levels.

The HPA axis is critical for the body's ability to respond to stress. Chronic stress can lead to dysregulation of the HPA axis, which can have negative effects on physical and mental health. For example, chronic stress can lead to increased cortisol levels, which can contribute to the development of cardiovascular disease, diabetes, and depression.

Our healthcare system is **clueless** to adrenal fatigue syndrome because:

- There is no ICD 10 code
- It's not taught in medical school
- It's not covered by insurance
- It affects greater than 70% of the population (from my clinical experience)
- It is treated with anti-depressants, steroids, or not at all
- The inflammatory response is the beginning of the immune response. Examples are stress, blood sugar, and trauma (physical and emotional). Inflammatory levels in turn drive the adrenals to exhaustion.

In summary, the HPA axis (see Figure 5.1) is a complex neuroendocrine system that plays a critical role in regulating the body's response to stress. It involves the hypothalamus, pituitary gland, and adrenal glands, which work together to release hormones that affect various physiological processes. The HPA axis is tightly regulated by a feedback system to maintain balance in the body, and dysregulation of the HPA axis can have negative effects on physical and mental health.

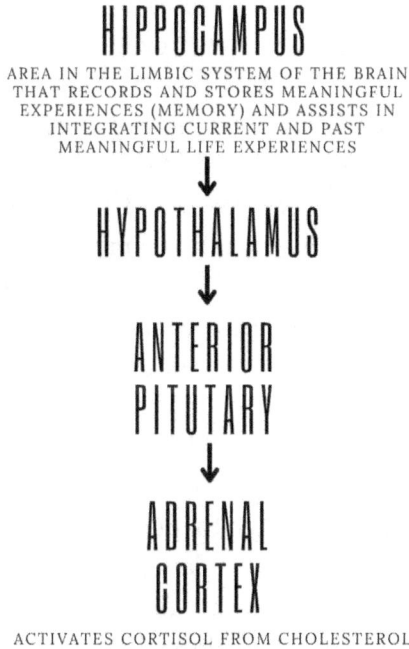

HIPPOCAMPUS

AREA IN THE LIMBIC SYSTEM OF THE BRAIN
THAT RECORDS AND STORES MEANINGFUL
EXPERIENCES (MEMORY) AND ASSISTS IN
INTEGRATING CURRENT AND PAST
MEANINGFUL LIFE EXPERIENCES

↓

HYPOTHALAMUS

↓

ANTERIOR PITUITARY

↓

ADRENAL CORTEX

ACTIVATES CORTISOL FROM CHOLESTEROL

Figure 5.1

Estrogen

Estrogen is a component of the endocrine pillar system that affects both women *and* men. Some breakthrough research on estrogen and its relationship with longevity and cancers has encouraged modern medicine to finally come around to acknowledging the medicinal benefits of cruciferous vegetables (such as kale, broccoli, Brussels sprouts, etc.).

New products like diindolylmethane (DIM) and indole-3-carbinol (13C) are hitting the market and making headlines in medical circles for their ability to reduce the risks of cancers related to elevated estrogen 2/16 hydroxy estrogen ratios. What's more, the easiest way to test levels of these estrogens (2/16s) is with a urine sample. Also, those same vegetables I mentioned above play a major role in liver and kidney detoxification through what is known as the cytochrome P450 pathway.

The medical establishment is now entrusting these cruciferous vegetables as precursors in the prevention of ovarian, uterine, breast, and prostate cancer. It is great news to finally see more info coming out on natural remedy and prevention, especially when you consider that the research and literature have been out for over 10 years now. Again, let me reiterate that positive symptoms of inflammatory prostate disorders are typically linked with elevated proinflammatory estrogens in the older male, not his testosterone, which often gets all the bad press concerning prostate issues.

On my website, an article titled *Senescence: The Art of Aging*, estrogen balance plays a major role as being a key player in the longevity of female lifespans. This is due in part to its role in eliminating stored toxic protein waste reserves in connective tissues. These toxic reserves are known to increase one's rate of senescence (a biological process that plays a key role in aging and age-related diseases) and death. Estrogens are found to have contra-effects in males when they are elevated above the maximum normal male levels, thus resulting in degenerative changes such as man-boobs, excessive fat accumulation, prostate issues, and premature death.

Telomeres

Telomeres are repeated segments of non-coding DNA that are attached to the ends of our chromosomes. They have been described as "tips on a pair of shoelaces." I like to think of them more like tiny antenna catching signals for chromosomes. Research shows that the shorter these tips on your chromosomes become, the shorter the life of the chromosome. This results in a shorter life for the cell and eventually a shorter life span for the host–you!

A major contributor to the destruction of our telomere lengths is inflammation (as found with cortisol release associated with stress, inflammatory diets, highly processed carbohydrates, and gluten consumption). Clinical depression and anxiety are also linked to shorter telomeres.

So, one of the keys to our overall health and longevity rests in maintaining your telomeres. Research has proven that restoring/

reversing shortened telomere lengths is possible through lifestyle changes like adequate rest, healthy diets, and reducing life's stresses. You can learn more about creating a better overall healthy diet, reducing life's stresses, and getting more rest in "Chapter 6: What Can I Do?"

There is great research revealed in the book *The Telomere Effect* by doctors Elizabeth Blackburn, Ph.D., and Elissa Epel, Ph.D. They write, "The research demonstrated how mothers of emotionally challenged children (like children diagnosed with autism), the physically impaired, and other debilitating diagnoses tended to have shorter telomeres than their chronologically same-aged peers. These shorter telomeres resulted in sluggish immune systems, increasing the possibilities of colds and infections." Obviously, these are afflictions that no caregiver has time to manage. And these extreme emotional states influence aging machinery in cells, namely your telomeres, mitochondria, and inflammatory processes.

So, to the life-altering caregivers, I truly cannot say, "I feel your stresses," since I have never had to walk a day in your shoes. I feel for you immensely, but I cannot say I know what it is like to feel your pain and sacrifice. Perhaps my heart is not large enough for such responsibility. I was given the opportunity to attempt to give back to my mother the love she blessed to me in the last year of her life as she struggled with COPD. However, I thankfully had the help of my siblings and the support of other family members whose lives she touched through her years.

I do know of the joy and stress that came with attempting to give back all the love she gave through her lifetime. But I am also quite certain that the lifetime caregiver stress threshold is at an entirely different level. So, though I cannot say "I feel your stresses," let me instead say "God bless you!" I do not want to think about what the world would be like without caregivers in it.

Please never stop searching until you find a doctor who understands the mind-body connection for your loved ones and your own special needs. One of my most cherished opportunities is when I receive the gift of working with patients who are caregivers. Please take time to exhale and focus on yourself, your adrenals, your nutrition, and your spirit. For as your prognosis goes, so goes the prognosis of those dependent on you. Take the time to tame your telomeres!

Bread

Here's a little ditty on one of America's favorite foods—bread—before we get into the entire food pyramid.

The glycemic food index measures the proximity of a food to pure glucose, which has a glycemic index of 100. The higher the glycemic number, the higher the glycemic load. And the higher the glycemic load, the quicker food turns to glucose (the measuring of blood-sugar levels in our bodies). An interesting example of some glycemic indexes or (G.I.) for foods are bananas (G.I. of 50), most candy bars (G.I. of 55), table sugar (G.I. of 60), and America's favorite whole wheat bread (G.I. of 71, a number that varies depending on the flour used).

That's correct—a slice of bread turns to sugar in the body faster than a candy bar. Think about that next time you're contemplating lunch. You're better off putting that turkey sandwich between two Mars bars than those slices of whole wheat bread. The National Institute of Health (NIH) didn't mention that in their food pyramid recommendation, did they? So maybe this obesity epidemic isn't solely caused by poor choices from consumers. Slick marketing and misinformation are everywhere. Making matters worse is that the NIH's new food pyramid, released in 2023, is even scarier than the one released in 1985.

That Pesky Pyramid

The reason grains are not recommended on my food pyramid anymore is because they are no longer a healthy food source (aside from the fresh-baked sourdough you might get at your local baker), mainly due to their high gluten contents, which promote inflammatory responses throughout the body. Many breads today are laced with substances called zorphines, which increase addiction responses.[4] Just like the

---

[4]   Pajak, Anjie. Metabolic IQ- Your Code to Health. Cosmo Health LTD, 2021. p. 154.

substance morphine, these chemicals cross the blood-brain barrier, creating an addiction response. This results in your craving the chemical and the product throughout the day. It's very much like what the Phillip Morris Company did with cigarettes back in the 1970s and 80s.

Glutens increase IBS, autoimmune disorders, and the glycemic index. The return on investment with grains for overall health is far too risky today, especially since 1985, when corporate wheat manufacturers changed the chemical structure of wheat to a GMO and increased the gluten content. Great substitutes for wheat are almond flour and cauliflower.

Since the American government began the NIH food pyramid in the early 1980s, obesity has skyrocketed by over 200%. Again, this coincides with the time wheat's structure was changed (genetically modified) to increase harvesting capabilities. Gluten content also increased, resulting in a 200% increase in autoimmune disorder diagnoses as well. Scary to think that there is a link in there somewhere.

Today's studies show that almost one out of every two (50%) of adults are obese, which has significant implications for public health.[5] That is an increase from around one in 10 back in the 1960s. Where is this trend going to put us in the next 40 years (if not before then)? Will everyone be obese? Not on my watch.

If these numbers were to have been changing at said rates 200 years ago, we would all be extinct by now. Think about this: In the 1960s and '70s, you could have run all the pharmaceutical commercials on a one-hour TV program. Today, you'll need a week's worth of primetime news hour programming to run their marketing campaigns. Have we really become that much sicker of a society in just 50 years? Don't answer! As I've said before, it's not that big pharma or the food congress is out to harm us per-se—but if you get in the way of their profits, you could become collateral damage.

---

[5] Hales, C. M., Carroll, M. D., Fryar, C. D., & Ogden, C. L. (2020). Prevalence of obesity and severe obesity among adults: United States, 2017–2018. NCHS Data Brief, no 360. National Center for Health Statistics.

Gut Problems

The #1 cause of most health problems starts with the gut. Whether the issue is physical, emotional, or hormonal, there is a direct impact on the gut. I like to say if you aren't having bowel movements every day, you have a gut problem. Period!

Toxic Food Metabolites and Mucoid Plaque

The danger of toxic food metabolites is that with a junk diet they can accumulate at too fast of a rate for the body to eliminate them. This condition is sometimes referred to as toxemia or acidosis.

Clogged colons are one of the major causes of disease today. For one, a clogged colon cannot efficiently absorb nutrients from the food it is processing. And for two, the moisture extracted from food as it is digested and the resultant mass can become gluey and adhesive, coating the walls of the colon and intestines. Modern processed foods are one of the main reasons for toxemia!

Estimates are that an average adult can have between seven to 25 pounds or more of layered impacted fecal matter clogging their digestive system. On average, a western citizen faithfully holds eight full meals of undigested food and waste matter in their digestive system at any one time!

That built-up decomposing material is a haven for germs and bacteria. They thrive at producing toxins that can enter the bloodstream and ultimately affect the entire body. The byproducts, including unstable oxidation elements (free radicals), damage our colon. This causes irritable bowel, Crohn's disease, and even colorectal cancer. For a measure of how serious this food-processing and corruption problem has become to western civilization, know this: **COLORECTAL CANCER IS INDEED CONSIDERED THE SECOND LEADING CAUSE OF CANCER-RELATED DEATHS IN THE INDUSTRIALIZED WORLD, AFTER LUNG CANCER!**[6]

---

[6] "Key Statistics for Colorectal Cancer." American Cancer Society, 13 Jan. 2023, www.cancer.org/cancer/colon-rectal-cancer/about/key-statistics.html.

12 MAJOR INDICATORS OF TOXICITY:

1. A constant feeling of sluggishness
2. Foggy head
3. Chronic fatigue
4. Susceptibility to infections (colds, flu, etc.)
5. Stomach and digestive problems
6. Bad breath
7. Bad body odor that persists after bathing
8. Poor wound healing
9. Chronic aches and pains
10. Suffering from a degenerative or inflammatory disease
11. Overweight
12. Expanded abdomen

Water and Our Metabolic Mayhem Connection

I know many of you won't like reading this, but … beware of your toxic showers, baths, and all uses of your municipal water sources. So-called heavy water, which is most of the unfiltered water used in our homes from city municipalities, contains high levels of fluoride, chlorine, and bromine. All of these are well-known toxins. Fluoride is even rated more toxic than lead. These are also three of the most toxic chemicals to the thyroid gland, breasts, and ovaries.

These three toxic chemicals share the same receptor sites, known as halogens, with life's essential mineral iodine. This is a key factor in multiple metabolic functions throughout the body. Halogen receptor sites are found highest in thyroid, breast, and ovarian tissues. Since most American diets fall far short of adequate iodine consumption, these receptor sites become inundated with toxic chemicals like fluoride, chlorine, and bromine—resulting in organ and tissue damage and disease.

Genetics

Genes turn on and off in response to their environments, diet, stress, and lifestyle choices. You are in control of most of your gene expressions, though. However, you are not off the hook when controlling your health and life—including your psychiatric conditions. Genes react to hormones such as insulin, cortisol, lepton, etc. They also react to foods, environmental conditions, and stress as seen in HPA axis suppression.

Epigenetics

The prefix "epi" means "over." So, the term "epigenetics" means those things that have an influence over our genes. A gene will not express itself unless the environment surrounding it becomes favorable to that expression. Both cellular DNA and chromatin modification (controlling gene expression) are influenced by our environment and play an important role in disease susceptibility. In simpler terms, it's not the genes themselves that predispose us to disease, but rather the things in our lives (i.e., diet, lifestyle, and environment) that act upon our genes. There is not a drug on this earth that regulates your genetic expressions greater or more powerfully than your diet and lifestyle. Yes, you are in more control than you know!

It's All in Our Genes ... or Is It?

It is commonly assumed—with no scientific basis—that if a condition "runs in the family" and appears in successive generations, that it must be genetic, right? But as I just said, genes are controlled by their environment—and without these environmental signals, they could not function.

Life experiences influence the function of our genes through epigenetics. So, we must ask why such narrow genetic assumptions are so widely embraced and enthusiastically accepted. Perhaps it is the neglect of developmental science or our tendency for a one-on-one causation for almost everything.

Life, in all its wonderful complexity, does not conform to such easy reductions. Perhaps it is a psychological escape that provides one with a powerful incentive to cling to genetically predisposed theories. We humans do not like feeling responsible for our own actions—or as a society for our failings.

If it could, genetics—the neutral, impersonal servant of nature—would relinquish us of our responsibilities and its ever-dark cloud of guilt. "It's all in the genes" is an explanation for the way things are that *will not threaten* the way things are. Succumbing to the all-too-common human urge to exonerate ourselves of responsibility, we as a culture have eagerly embraced the fundamentalism of a genetic predisposition. Truth be told, nothing is irreversibly dictated in our genes, and in reality, there is much that can be done in controlling our destiny towards radiant health.

Take the Challenge

There are many different factors that can negatively affect our health, vitality, and longevity over time, including:

- **Age:** There are many things we can do to prevent premature aging and fight the typical aging process. If you need proof, look around to see the differences in how some age versus others.
- **Genetics:** Yes, our genetic makeup can influence risks of developing diseases that impact your health and longevity. However, influence is not a determinate.
- **Lifestyle factors:** Poor diet, lack of exercise, smoking, and excessive alcohol consumption can all contribute to the deterioration of our health over time.
- **Environmental factors:** We all know that there are certain environmental factors that can have negative impacts on our health.
- **Stress:** As mentioned, this can have numerous effects on your health, including inflammation and a weakened immune system, which can contribute to many other diseases and illnesses down the road.

- **Lack of sleep:** Insufficient sleep can also weaken immunity and increase the risk of developing chronic health issues.
- **Medical conditions:** Chronic medical conditions such as heart disease, diabetes, and autoimmune disorders contribute to the deterioration of your health.

There are more solutions that will be shared later in this book, but in the meantime, focus on what is going into your mouth and how often, moving whenever you think about it, and doing the work to take an active role in your stress management.

Your Reflection Corner

Chapter 5: How Did This Happen?

You are on a health journey. It is time to discover more about yourself before you continue reading. Consider the following questions to begin your healing and prevention journey:

1. Do you identify with any of the scenarios or health issues described in this chapter?
2. What are your symptoms? When did they start? How severe would you rate them? Describe them in full detail.
3. If you had these issues before, how did you treat them? What was and was not successful about this treatment?
4. Has anything new happened in your life or environment that may have sparked this change?
5. Were there any recent changes to your diet, exercise routine, or medication regimen that could be contributing to your symptoms?
6. Are you experiencing any other health conditions that could be contributing to the symptoms?
7. Do you have any family history of health issues?

By knowing more about yourself, you can continue to be informed in order to take your best pathway forward. Next, we will discuss solutions to the pesky causes of your less-than-optimal health.

Do You Know?

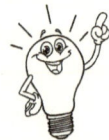

Pearl: Vino? But, of Course

Drinking red wine can increase longevity. Red wine contains a nutrient called resveratrol; a powerful antioxidant known to activate a certain class of anti-aging gene known as sirtuins. These genes, referred to as SIRT-1 longevity genes, are found to be abundant in healthy centurions (those who live to 100 years old and older). How much red wine is needed? A lot. So, consider a little red wine and supplementation with 1,000 mg per day of resveratrol. Supplements are best in the morning; save the wine for the evening.

CHAPTER 6

WHAT CAN I DO?

IF YOU DO NOTHING ELSE for yourself today, at least honor your body as the temple that it is for you. You only get this one body in life, no do-overs. It can either serve you or cripple you. If you let your health continue to spiral in an unhealthy way, disease and debilitation are surely in your future.

Trust me. I have seen patient after patient willing to do anything to have a better life AFTER their health has already started to deteriorate. Some of them make amazing changes, but others sadly passed a point of no return. Others still don't have the energy to make the changes required, because the abuse inflicted on their body made it where there was not much left for them to draw upon. Don't become a medical nightmare! Become a health ambassador!

Look, bad health habits could literally be costing you your life. As I write this, I think of my friends who have died far too early in life. Oh, how I wish I could have had more time with them. I also think of my patients, who I wish I could have met earlier and helped on their journey back to better health. Who do you know that declined to care for themselves and met a needless, premature death?

The stakes are high when it comes to your diet and physical fitness! If you don't grab control of your health today, you are possibly setting your life up for one of disease, whether it's cardiovascular, type 2 diabetes, cancer, or respiratory disease. Is that how you want to spend your golden years? Instead, you could live like you did in your earlier years into your retirement: golfing, weight training, enjoying the beach, biking, playing tennis, and more.

Starting today, be your own health champion! You can do this!

Humans Do What They Value

It has been said you can tell how much someone actually values something by how much time they invest in it. Humans do what they value, not what they say they value. What are you saying about how you value your health? How much time per day/week is spent respecting your values toward your health? It is not about what you say you do or what you are going to do. Time spent tells the truth about what value you place on everything. Is your health even worth 20 minutes of exercise a day? What about three healthy meals? Is your health worth that?

The Basics

Get back to the basics: "Basics" being the things you do every day, day-in and day-out, month-in and month-out, year-in and year-out. When you have good basics, you can get away with occasional indulgence. You know what you can do in many areas of your life to have better health outcomes, so start there.

We all know to do the following:

- **Start moving.** Some form of movement is critical. After all, life is motion.
- **Start eating for energy.** We all know that if your diet is a disaster, your health will soon be the same.
- **Start paying attention to your body's needs**. Drink more water if you are constantly thirsty. Consider being more active if you are tired all the time—and get checked out to see if something else is going on.
- **Avoid unhealthy behaviors.** Smoking and excessive alcohol can feel good in the moment, but they are also disastrous for your health.
- **Take deliberate action to manage your stress.** There are easy things you can do like take a walk in nature every day, mediate, journal, and spend time with God.

- **Focus on healthy sleep habits.** Yes, this is a big one! Get no less than seven hours of quality sleep!
- **Find positive people.** And then surround yourself with them.

My solutions, which I have developed by working for over 30 years on my basics and the basics of my patients, are in the next chapter, Solutions. But first, I wanted to give you a taste of what you already know and where you could get started today.

Responsibility and Control

You can never give responsibility away. The only thing you can give away is control. And the law of control states: You only feel good about yourself to the degree to which you are in control over your life.

You are always completely responsible. So, in giving up control, you're giving up your peace of mind. Some give control away to their medical doctors and pharmaceutical companies, while others make decisions as to what is best for them. Others still give up their control by just giving up altogether, releasing all discipline and responsibility of their own health outcomes. Then there are those who trust that they have bad genes and think their best outcomes are the outcomes of those before them—WRONG!

No matter how you give up your control, you will suffer. You must invest in your health in the same way you invested in your children, career, favorite car, or most enjoyable hobby. If you take the time to learn about your body and how to take care of it, you will reap rewards beyond your imagination. Your body is an incredible machine that can endure only so much neglect, but it can achieve incredible things with the right investment.

Personal Investment

Investing in change is a chosen priority. To succeed, you need an end result in mind. All of us need to determine where we choose to invest our time—X, Y, or Z. Either we invest our time in diet, exercise, and weight loss, or we will be investing in fending off high blood pressure, diabetes, or some other metabolic disease.

You must prioritize your schedule accordingly to maximize your results. It may be that you need more exercise time or to invest more time in planning and implementing a healthier diet. You may need some more injury recovery time, or maybe you just need to maximize how your time is spent by prioritizing your planning. Most people fail to maximize their outcome due to lack of organization or a lack of knowledge of how to prioritize their time and energy into a daily routine.

Many people get overwhelmed trying to focus on everything all at once. When they do, it makes it easier to fail. Getting healthy comes in stages. Sometimes we may need a coach to get us through certain stages, like planning out our journey to better health and wellness. A coach can help us understand the best steps to take to get started in a way that will make us more likely to prevail. For instance, we may want to go all in, but our coach may suggest that we fix one stage before moving on to another. For example, we may need to fix a stomach issue before addressing weight loss issues or work on weight loss before implementing a new exercise routine.

There are key areas that can set you up for success, so planning before you start can help your outcomes. For instance:

- Who you surround yourself with and choose in your support group is crucial. For example, it is easier to quit drinking beer if you surround yourself with people who don't drink.
- It is easier to get to the gym or yoga if it is just down the street.
- It is easier to keep your chiropractic or therapy visits if they are local.
- It is easier to be successful with your goals if you hang around inspiring, successful, goal-oriented, likeminded people.
- It is also easier to have a negative outlook with negative results if you are hanging in a negative environment. So, conversely, if you hang around with positive people, you will have more positive thoughts, which will help you get further in your goals.

There is a saying: "Keep it simple, stupid." Let's drop the stupid part, though, and just say, "Keep it simple." Decide first where you need to start your journey. Don't forget to ask for a little help from your higher power for guidance and support. If you feel you will be more successful in developing your schedule and meeting your needs with a Life Coach, go to www.DrJoeyJones.com. As you know, this is an area of passion for me, so I would love nothing more than to go on this journey with you!

Choose Your Doctor Wisely

Size up your doctor. Do they fit the model you are looking for physically, mentally, and spiritually? Is their resume up to date? They are your coach, sometimes your life coach. Did they pass the interview? They are not your mommy or daddy; you were not born into their care or a relationship with them. Choose diligently. It is your hire, not theirs. Do they walk *your* walk and talk *your* talk? Do they look like the model of health for which you are trying to be? Do they respect your opinion? After all, it is your life that matters.

Three major life changing decisions are made in most people's lifetimes: whom you marry (which is hopefully forever), the career you choose (choose wisely, it is your livelihood), and the doctor who cares for you (your life may depend on it). It is not about who is in your insurance network—it's about who is going to help you make critical health decisions as you age.

Again, too much authority tends to be given to someone in a white coat. By giving yourself or a loved one's health over to an authority figure, you are becoming a victim twice. Choosing your perfect health care <u>team</u> can mean the difference between thriving, or just surviving. So, choose your team's physician carefully. God bless you if you are limited to only someone in your insurance network, especially if there are few choices locally. I'm sorry! Your life is worth more than limitations set by your insurance plan.

Patient Accountability Act:
Investing in One's Health

One thing every person does have 100% investment responsibility for is their health. You should also have 100% say in control of your outcome concerning your health—unlike investing in the financial market or the lottery, where you are relying on someone else to produce results for your hard work and investment.

You cannot rely on or put the outcome of your life and body's health in the hands of the prescription pad salespeople or the physician chosen from the list of your insurance carrier demands. You must take responsibility to educate yourself about your priceless investment—your health—to guarantee the absolute best R.O.I. possible.

Remember: With knowledge comes power. With power comes strength. With strength comes self-control and self-respect. The truly wealthiest are the healthiest.

Now, let's gain some more knowledge regarding supplementation.

Choosing the Right Supplements

The key here is that it's better to pay a little more for <u>something</u> than to pay anything for nothing. Avoid wasting your money on inferior products sold on TV. One of my long-standing jokes is, "If they are selling it on TV, don't buy it." You never see a broccoli commercial on television, do you? The good stuff sells itself. Same goes for commercial health food stores and chain store pharmacies with their poor-quality fake vitamins.

Learn how to detect tall tale signs of "parts is parts" vitamins, also known as vitamers or isolates. These are not natural products even if they are produced from organic substances like coal tar and limestone. Since they are not of the same structure as foods found in nature, the body often cannot utilize them. In fact, the body may even become depleted of other essential nutrients trying to utilize synthetic vitamin substitutes.

Synthetic vitamins are chemically different and inferior to natural mixtures found in organic vitamins, which always contain synergistic mineral counterparts. So, once again, the sad truth is that most of the popular vitamins sold on TV are too good to be true. It is the same for most supplements sold at popular pharmacies and health food stores—they are synthetic vitamins or vitamers and isolates.

So, here is how to read a label, what to look for in a good vitamin, and what to avoid in suboptimal vitamer and isolates. Start with organically based whole food supplements whenever possible, as these set the industrial standards for authenticity and potency. Look for these tall tale signs of insufficiencies when reading supplement labels:

- **Calcium**: Often sold as calcium carbonate, this is limestone. You might as well lick a rock. Calcium must be ionized to be functional in the body, which this is not. In fact, it's far from it. Calcium carbonate = a metal-based vitamin. That is not good.
- **Magnesium Oxide**: Oxide is also metal-based, which means the body cannot break it down, therefore it cannot be used. These are the kind of supplements that upset most people's stomachs.
- **Vitamin C**: This is sold as ascorbic acid. If you see this ... run! Ascorbic acid is not a vitamin; it is only 5% of the vitamin C complex. You cannot sell someone a tire and call it a car. Nothing in nature comes in 500mg or 1,000mg. This means it is not natural. It won't even fight off the common cold, because it is only the antioxidant component of vitamin C.
- **Vitamin E**: This is often sold as alpha-tocopherol or d-alpha. Again ... no! Just return it. It is a synthetic isolate, or a vitamer much like vitamin C's ascorbic acid. It is the antioxidant portion of the vitamin only. It is void of all the other tocopherols and other constituents, like selenium, that make up the whole vitamin as it is found in nature. Sold as an isolate like this, as it most often is, can lead to sterility issues.
- **Glucosamine**: This one is sold as glucosamine HCL. Again, it's an isolate. Look for your glucosamine in sulfate form— that is the sulfur component that contains the medicinal properties.

These are a few signs of synthetic vitamins and isolates, or fractions of vitamin compounds. These isolates function more like a drug in the body and will often deplete you of nutrients. Organic vitamins contain minerals. Organic minerals contain vitamins. This is the way nature works. You are a gift of nature, so it only makes sense that this is the way your body works.

There are some critical vitamin supplements that I feel compelled to share more particulars on below, starting with:

Calcium

There is more calcium in the human body than all other minerals combined, so it makes sense that there are more calcium supplements sold than any other mineral. The key to calcium use is quality of assimilation, not quantity ingested. Sadly, quite often the most popular calcium products on the market are non-absorbable by our bodies and are about as useful to our health as licking the sidewalk.

Our bodies use calcium to aid in the prevention of osteoporosis, arthritic diseases, immune system boosters, and much more. Calcium must be in the ionized form for maximum assimilation. To become ionized, an electrical charge must be gained. If it is not ionized, it will not be assimilated for use. The problem is that most calcium comes in carbonate form.

Carbonates are very difficult for the body to use; they require multiple steps before they become ionized for absorption in the body. Carbonates are a product of limestone—again, you might as well be licking the sidewalk. Carbonate calcium products require high amounts of hydrochloric acid for assimilation and high levels of digestive enzymes to break them down.

Two by-products, HCl and digestive enzymes, are lacking in optimal amounts in most people's digestive systems to begin with due to poor diet choices. Look for highly absorbable forms of calcium like calcium lactate, calcium citrate, or some type of similar highly acidic base calcium. Why? Because these forms require very few enzymatic steps to reach their ionized form of calcium. The form of calcium utilized and absorbed from our GI tract is calcium bicarbonate. The faster the conversion of calcium products to calcium bicarbonate, the better.

The role of vitamin D in calcium assimilation is that of picking up calcium from the gut and putting it in the blood to later be distributed in the tissue via vitamin F (perhaps better known as polyunsaturated fatty acids like fish oils, flaxseed, etc.). The key players in the assimilation and absorption of calcium lie in the role of these polyunsaturated fatty acids. They transport calcium from the blood to the tissue, bones, etc. Kidney stones, osteoporosis, cataracts, and calcium accumulation in arteries are all signs of poor calcium absorption and polyunsaturated fatty acid deficiencies. I'm not referring to an excess of calcium ingestion—again, it is a lack of calcium utilization.

Another important factor in calcium absorption is its role in the function of white blood cells when an infection occurs in the body. Adequate serum calcium levels are necessary for optimal function of white blood cells locating infections (this is known as the calcium wave effect). In both osteoporosis and osteopenia, prevention lies in the assimilation and utilization of calcium and its bone-building counterparts. (The key here is bone strength, not bone density.) Here lies my problem with bone density testing and the use of bisphosphonate drugs for treatment of bone density issues such as osteopenia.

Bone health requires the orchestrated turnover of bone. Bisphosphonate drugs inhibit the osteoclastic process, resulting in increased body density, but do nothing to improve bone strength. And we haven't even mentioned the horrific complications seen only with bisphosphonates, such as osteonecrosis (i.e., bone death), which is the rotting of the jaw bones and weakening of weight-bearing bones like the femur.

So, to prevent osteoporosis, think of bone strengthening supplements and exercises (weight-bearing exercises are best). Additionally, try supplementation with highly absorbable (preferably plant-based) calcium products and their synergistic counterparts (minerals like magnesium, boron, vitamin C, vitamin D, and others).

*Calcium: the key is in assimilation, not ingestion.

Some **clinical signs** of calcium deficiencies include:

- Leg cramps, predominantly in your lower legs (worse at night). For this, think calcium and magnesium supplementation.
- Growing pains in children due to low calcium reserves in tissue (not able to meet the demand for growing bones). Milk does not work here! Instead, think about using plant-based calcium supplementations.

Little Ditty about Magnesium

Magnesium controls over 300 enzyme reactions in the body and brain. Magnesium insufficiency or deficiency is common in people who consume high carbohydrate diets. A loss of magnesium is often seen in blood sugar surges, cortisol surges, and elevated insulin and in cases of stress, anxiety, and depression, all of which are common elements in today's society. Magnesium deficiency is also a common side effect of most medications, perhaps none more so than antacids and acid blockers. So, it's no surprise that magnesium deficiencies or insufficiencies are at epidemic proportions today thanks to a vast array of dietary, environmental, and social stressors like never before in history.

Magnesium, as with most minerals, helps us to regulate our parasympathetic nervous system for relaxation and digestion. Sadly, our lives today are being overrun by our fight, flight, or freeze response of the sympathetic nervous system, leaving many of us with the difficulty or inability to calm down. A common example of this is the difficulty so many people are having falling asleep, which has led to mass prescriptions for sleep medications—most of which are very addictive and difficult to discontinue.

Magnesium deficiencies are common in those with depression, anxiety, ADD, and ADHD. Again, these are symptoms of weak parasympathetic nervous system function. Sadly, to make conditions worse, most of the medications used to treat these disorders are major contributors to magnesium depletion.

The inadequate daily intake of plant materials and consumption of processed food with poor nutritional contents helps contribute to magnesium deficiency.[7]

Historical nutritional data for developed countries suggest that produce (especially vegetables), has experienced as high as a 40 percent decline in mineral, vitamin, and protein content over the last century.[8]

Therefore, obtaining magnesium and minerals and trace elements from nutrition rich plants remains critical for reaching adequate daily intake of these mineral nutrients.[9]

To recap, magnesium is one of the most overlooked and most depleted minerals in our diets today. Deficiencies can lead to high blood pressure, anxiety, depression, muscular tension and spasms, impaired liver and brain function, cancer, heart disease, and sleep disturbances. For the best results when supplementing and for best absorption, look for plant-based, organic forms like magnesium lactate or citrate. (FYI, magnesium oxide, found in many of the commercialized brands, is not well tolerated and commonly causes loose stools and digestive disturbances.) Magnesium is best absorbed in 150-250 mg doses two to three times per day.

The following disorders are commonly associated with a magnesium deficiency:

- Arrythmia
- Asthma
- ADD/ADHD
- Anxiety
- Auto immune disorders
- Constipation
- Depression
- Gut disorders like colitis, Crohn's, and peptic ulcers
- High blood pressure

---

[7] Standard Process E-Z Mg: 4. Rosanoff, A. Plant and Soil 2013, 368 (1-2), 139-153.
[8] Standard Process E-Z Mg: 5. Davis, D. R. HortScience 2009, 44 (1).
[9] Standard Process E-Z Mg: 6. Nielsen, F. H., Crop and Pasture Science 2015, 66 (12).

- Hypoglycemia
- Insomnia
- Kidney stones
- Headaches
- Muscle cramps
- PMS
- Syndrome-X
- Tremors
- Insulin resistance and obesity (due to high carbohydrate diets)

Prebiotics/Probiotics vs. Antibiotics

Antibiotics means "anti-life" and are designed to eliminate dangerous pathogens from our bodies. However, their usage destroys both our bad and good bacteria. This results in very compromised natural immune systems, as the antibiotics attack our inborn defense systems within our gut flora. Prebiotic and probiotic supplementation helps us restore, rebuild, and maintain our supporting gut flora, thus maintaining a healthy gut environment to protect against our next infectious threat. Probiotics help us support bowel consistency and regularities and improve digestion, absorption, and elimination. Probiotics are a key adjunct to anyone's antibiotic therapy.

Prebiotics are the new kid on the block. These are a specific form of bacteria in which we all have our own personal strains unique to our inherited genomes from our parents' intestinal flora. Thus, these prebiotics fuel our native microbes, powerfully supporting our immune systems. Most prebiotics thrive on non-digestible fibers from sources like chicory root and even sweet potatoes. These sources are broken down and absorbed by our colonic bacteria, which are unique to our own gene-specific, good gut bacteria.

When I begin someone on a new vitamin, mineral, or herbal protocol, I let them know we are trying them out on a new chemistry to the body. Same goes for a new medication. I highly recommend they tell their family and those whose opinion they respect to let them know if they notice any changes in behavior during onset of protocol use.

Some of Dr. J's Favorite Supplements and Why

- Vitamin B Complex
  - An important adjunct to slowing the progression of most all degenerative and debilitating diseases
  - Nerve integrity and cell energy reactions
  - Carbohydrate metabolism, oxidation of lactic acid

The energy that a cell needs to maintain itself and perform its various functions is supplied by the oxidation of the food within the cell. In this respect, vitamin B complex performs an important role by catalyzing the various chain reactions through its co-enzymes. This to a very large extent is related to carbohydrates' metabolism, and as such the requirements for vitamin B vary according to the amounts of carbohydrates ingested, particularly sugars.

- Chlorophyll
  - Increases platelet counts, which are concerned with the elimination of protein tissue toxic debris that accumulate in tissue fluids. Benefits include:
  - Improves blood purification
  - Prevents nerve atrophy
  - Increases vitamins A, E, K, and F (essential fatty acids)
  - Increases real blood count

- CoQ10
  - Increases cellular oxidation (highest concentrations found in cell mitochondria). Mitochondria are high in fatty acid substances (EFAs), nucleoproteins, and phospholipids.
  - Vital for energy production
  - Antioxidant protects cell from negative byproducts and free radicals
  - Critical in brain health
  - Destroyed by statin (cholesterol lowering) drug use

- Cruciferous Vegetable
  - Supports phases I and II liver and kidney detoxification through the cytochrome P450 enzyme system obtained from vegetables, such as kale and Brussels sprouts
  - Maintains normal liver function
  - Highest concentration of phytonutrients
  - High in antioxidant activity
  - Helps neutralize free radicals, which can lead to cancers
  - Support healthy eye function

- Choline (methyl group)
  - Lipotropic factor
  - Promotes the elimination of proteins associated with senescence along with lecithin (EFA) and phosphorus
  - 95% of the plasma phospholipids contain choline
  - Decrease in liver phosphatides with diet deficient in choline
  - Both kidney and liver lesions result from choline deficiencies due to failure of phospholipid synthesis

- DHEA
  - This is the superstar of super hormones and one of the most powerful tools available for enhancing and extending life. Produced in the adrenal glands, it's metabolized into androstenedione, which is converted directly into testosterone. Precursor to most all hormones, both male and female.
  - Decreases with age ... by age 40 we have about half of what we had in our 20s
  - Increased feeling of energy and well-being
  - Improved insulin sensitivity and glucose tolerance
  - Decreases coronary heart disease
  - Decreases obesity
  - Slows progression of arteriosclerosis
  - Enhanced libido and erectile ability

- Reduced depression
- Improved cognitive function

- Lecithin
  - Key component in phospholipid formation, which is necessary for protein debris elimination. Antagonist to cholesterol due to phospholipids opposing the influence of cholesterol. Because phospholipids offer "sheathing" layers between which cholesterol and proteins are held, cholesterol is rendered harmless.
  - High concentration found in eggs
  - Deficiencies result in protein metabolism interference
  - Phospholipid precursor

- Iodine
  - An EFA/iodine balance is essential for the health and vitality of every tissue in the body
  - Iodine and thyroid are utilized in the EFA transfer reaction of the lipoprotein protein molecule in the liver
  - Key link in the biochemistry of the "sheathing" material responsible for removing toxic protein debris out of the body
  - Predisposes an important component in all thyroid functions
  - Receptor sites in the body are blocked by chlorine, fluorine, and bromine exposure

- Manganese
  - Enhances support to the anterior pituitary gland and its modulation of hormones
  - Precursor in the Krebs (energy) cycle
  - Mineral factor necessary for pituitary activity

- Vitamin E
  - Increases tissue oxidation (oxygen carrying capability)
  - Precursor to sex hormones

- Antioxidant
- Retards the development of cancers by influence of cell maturation and differentiation
- Involved in the protective association (much like vitamin A of protein with lipid sheathing)

- Vitamin A
  - Protects against protein cellular debris activity with lipoids in developing (catalyzing) protective sheathing materials with EFAs like vitamin F in the elimination of toxins from our bodies, etc.
  - Powerful antioxidant, anti-inflammatory, anti-cancerous properties
  - Beneficial in arthritis, iodine utilization, burn treatments, cancer, and lecithin metabolism
  - Deficiency can lead to sterility like that of vitamin E
  - Platelet counts diminished in vitamin A deficiency

- Thymus
  - Promotes a youthful epidermis (so called thymic complexion) possibly due to its activity in promoting the protective association of proteins with lipoids
  - Thymus extract and choline as well as other methyl groups act as anti-carcinogens
  - T-cell producer
  - Aids in antibody production
  - Immune system enhancer

- RNA
  - The nucleic acid of the cytoplasm
  - RNA is the growth promoter when added to tissue
  - Associated with protein synthesis and cell division
  - Supports growth by activating protein synthesis memory factor of the cell
  - Promotes healing
  - Aids in memory support

Exercise

Exercise is any activity that will make you stronger, help you lose body fat, improve cardiovascular performance, improve endurance and flexibility, and build you up by improving bone density and muscle mass. Exercise is designed to build you up, not break you down. Personally, I find high-intensity, short duration, weight resistance exercise most favorable for fast results with minimal injury. There are undoubtedly physical benefits in many other forms of exercise such as tennis, running (treadmills), golf, basketball, baseball, racquetball, soccer, and more. But in addition to the pleasurable benefits that come from these activities, they also come with many risks such as knee, ankle, elbow, shoulder, and back injuries.

Perhaps even the least physical of all, golf, will send 7 out of 10 golfers to health professionals each year.[10] Don't even get me started on running related injuries like bad knees, shin splints, plantar fasciitis, and back and hip injuries. Many injuries arise from the continuous, punishing blows upon foot impact of three times one's body weight in each step. That is about 120 tons of collective force per mile for a 150-lb. runner.

So, if you are heavier and are thinking about running as an activity to get in shape or lose weight, you might want to seriously reconsider losing the weight first. Injuries equal setbacks, and if you're attempting these activities to get healthier, you've defeated the purpose. Again, much like caring for an expensive, high-performance automobile or thoroughbred racehorse, preparation, rest, recovery, and all things in moderation are the keys to success in longevity.

What about cardiovascular health and endurance? Everyone knows you must perform long, boring, monotonous activities to improve heart and lung health, right? So, we need treadmills, stair

---

[10] (2018, January 31). Sports Injury Statistics Suggest: Golf is More Dangerous than Rugby. Golf Support. https://golfsupport.com/blog/sports-related-injuries-golf-more-dangerous-than-rugby/#:~:text=Injuries%20in%20Golf%20are%20Much%20More%20Common%20than%20Widely%20Believed&text=In%20professionals%2C%20the%20incidence%20rates,least%20once%20in%20a%20lifetime

climbers, running, biking, and walking, right? Surprisingly, the answer is no.

People often mistake cardiovascular fitness and endurance workouts as the same thing. But they are not the same. The heart and lungs do not become stronger from running or any other form of strenuous fitness—certainly not from the infamous aerobic exercises like jogging, swimming, or biking. As Fredrick Hahn explains in his book, *The Slow Burn Fitness Revelation*, while a person who decides to start taking the stairs up to their fourth-floor apartment might be initially fatigued, this will improve. Continuing to take the stairs will make it easier to get to the fourth floor as the weeks progress.

But it's the strength of our leg, hip, and back muscles that are better able now to utilize oxygen, thus taking the strain off the heart and lungs. Stronger muscles work more efficiently to draw oxygen from the blood, thus reducing demand on the heart and lungs, which gives the impression of improved cardiovascular and cardiopulmonary fitness. The point I am getting to here is that by strengthening your body's muscles, they can function within the capacity of your heart and lungs. The single most effective and least time-consuming way to strengthen one's body at any age is weight resistant strength training.

The purpose of exercise is to build you up, not beat you up.

Physical Health 101

I think we all know the things we can do to become a better and healthier version of ourselves, so much of the material in here may be a repeat for you. Yet, we all need continual reminders to get us back on the right track for optimal and radiant health for the long haul. Here is what keeps me on track:

- Regular exercise (short duration/high-intensity workouts)
- Maintaining blood sugar balance
- Eating a protein sufficient diet
- Limiting alcohol intake (nothing for me, but keep yours mild)
- Resting seven to nine hours per night

- Detoxing daily (systemic detox through supplementation if sweating isn't possible)
- Releasing dopamine through healthy choices, and doing so often
- Maintain a healthy gut (i.e., bowel movements, one per day minimum)

FIT

I prioritize high-intensity exercises of short duration. After all, less time-consuming means more compliance. It's easy to implement into one's schedule, so there's no excuse for not having enough time. Remember the definition of exercise (not yoga). Though yoga is great, it typically does not fit the definition of "build you up." For more information on exercising and routines, visit www.drjoeyjones.com.

Recommended Blood Tests

- **Homocysteine:** Can indicate if you are likely to have a heart attack or stroke. Levels of homocysteine can be lowered with folic acid, B6, and B12. B vitamin deficiencies are common when taking a wide range of drugs, from aspirin to estrogens to stomach acid suppressors (Nexium and Prilosec), which interfere with B vitamin metabolism. Elevated risk of homocysteine levels includes Parkinson's, Alzheimer's, heart disease, and vascular dementia. Homocysteine is an amino acid that is produced in the body, and B vitamins are your best protection against elevated levels.
  - Normal levels – Around 10 mg/dL

- **C-Reactive Protein** (High sensitivity): Measures inflammation factors in arteries. Studies indicated that C-reactive protein may be the most accurate risk factor predicting a heart attack and stroke. The higher the level of CRP, the greater the likelihood that your body is being harmed by inflammation. More enlightened physicians are offering this test. If your physician does not, you should request it or change doctors.

- ○ <u>Normal levels</u> – Below 3 mg/dL

- **Fibrinogen:** High levels of this blood clotting factor increase the risk of heart attack and stroke.
- **DHEA-Sulfate:** Produced mainly in the adrenal glands. DHEA is a direct precursor of most steroid hormones, and perhaps one of the most powerful tools for enhancing and extending life.
- **PSA (Prostate Specific Antigen):** Can provide early warning signs for prostate disorders, including cancer.
- **Free Testosterone:** Most reliable test for determining whether testosterone replacement should be considered as a therapy for low testosterone, depression, abdominal obesity, poor mental performance, or loss of libido.
- **Estradiol:** For women and men (determines the proper amount in the body).
- **CBC/Chemistry Profile:** *Most popular test. Measures over 35 different blood components including cholesterol, iron, triglycerides, glucose, blood cell counts, minerals, liver, and kidney function, etc.
- **A1C Test** (Hemoglobin A1C or HbA1C): Measures average blood sugar over the past three months. Helps determine diagnosis of prediabetes and diabetes.
- Normal range – Below 5.7%
- **Coenzyme Q10:** One of the best antioxidants for the heart. They keep your mitochondria working.
- **Insulin Fasting:** Helps determine resistance (sensitivity). A pre-diabetic state, and sugar handling problems.
- **Thyroid Panel:** First test for overall thyroid function (TSH, T4, Free T3).
- **Insulin Panel:** HOMA-IR stands for homeostatic model assessment of insulin resistance. It marks both the presence and extent of any insulin resistance that you might currently express. It is a terrific way to identify between your baseline

(fasting) blood sugar and the response to insulin (your insulin resistance score). A healthy range to aim for is 1.0.

Dr. J's Protocol for Stress Management and Nutritional Support of Adrenal Fatigue Syndrome

I recommend the following: adrenal gland-specific targeting herbs, hypothalamus gland cytosol extract, whole food B-complex vitamins, and pituitary, adrenal, and thyroid nuclei protein extract supplements.

As for diet modifications, aim for: Gluten-free, low glycemic, parasympathetic, and sympathetic nervous system supplementation to help manage your stress response.

Visit my website for more detailed information regarding a good diet and supplements to seek out.

Take Action:

Chronic stress breaks down both adrenal and pancreas function, and stress and anxiety constantly bombard your body with adrenalin, making you nervous and tense. The elevated adrenals signal your pancreas to increase insulin secretion, resulting in blood sugar problems and eventually pancreatic burnout. This ultimately pushes the body towards hypoglycemia and other sugar handling problems like obesity and type II diabetes, (not to mention the not so flattering tire-around-the-waist look.)

But I have good news! There are several actions you can take to help your body cope while you strengthen your adrenal and nervous system.

Getting Started:

Avoid prescription drugs whenever possible. Use only as a last or temporary resort. Examples are anti-anxiety drugs (i.e., Xanax, Klonopin, etc.) and sleep aids (i.e., Ambien), which can become addictive and have undesirable side effects.

Find a doctor who evaluates adrenal function using Adrenal Stress Index (ASI) saliva testing and who comprehends HPA axis regulation and adrenal hormone balancing. This protocol has been a life changer for hundreds of my patients. It's been said that as go your adrenals, so goes you. Just about every autonomic disorder diagnosis holds some relationship with stress and its connection to inflammation and elevated cortisol levels.

Nearly every patient in my practice with a diagnosis of an autoimmune disorder responded remarkably well with adrenal support therapy. Perhaps one of the saddest medical blunders to our society today is that adrenal fatigue is not being taught in medical schools. Because adrenal fatigue issues do not have a billing code number in the system, physicians cannot get reimbursed for billing adrenal-related charges. Given the amount of stress occurring in our lives today, it is mind-blowing that our healthcare system does not place more focus on it.

Rejoice in Your Breath!

Go to your breath. That is where you will find your inner self. Life lives in the breath. Go to the breath, and you will be in the moment. All life, at any given moment, your breath can calm you. Hold on to each breath for a moment, letting it go slowly. Exhale for one second longer than you inhale. You can never get back a breath, nor obtain one that has not yet arrived. Therefore, in that breath you are always living in the moment. When the mind wanders, or things seem out of your control, stay with your breath. You can live for weeks without food, days without water, but only minutes without breath.

> *"Time does not wait for any man and breathing out is no guarantee for breathing in again."*
> Master Yunmen

Time to Get Serious!

Taking your health seriously can be the most important thing you ever do. This one step can create an impact that spans across every area of your life and those around you. Yes, it is hard to take steps to create new habits and stop old behaviors that you may have had your entire adult life. However, you only get one life and one body. If you take care of that one body, it will take care of you.

There are so many benefits to taking care of our bodies, including feeling like you could run through a brick wall and having energy like the energizer bunny, confidence like the incredible hulk, and the optimism of Tony Robbins. There are many more positive impacts, such as improved quality of sleep. Let's face it, we could all use some extra quality zzz's in our lives to improve our mood and overall well-being.

If you commit to investing in yourself, the return on your investment is immeasurable. One benefit will lead to another and another and another, until your entire life is rocking! Then, the impact your positively incredible life has on others will only be compounded by the positive influence they have on those around them. You see, you can create a health wave throughout the United States and the rest of the world—just by investing in yourself. That may sound crazy, but I believe it to be true!

By making a few key changes, other changes will follow until you find yourself in a totally different reality. Don't start too big, but do commit and take action. If you go too big, that can overwhelm you and keep you from persevering. Small efforts can compound. The key is to admit that you need to make changes in your life, commit to them, and then go after a better life for yourself! A new body and positive mental health are waiting for you around the corner. Start today!

Healthcare Reform vs. Health Reform

Americans don't need "healthcare" reform, we need "health" reform. As I've said, Americans don't have a healthcare system; we have a sick care system. Healthcare reform will not reform health care by itself. Only by becoming healthy individuals can we reform our healthcare system. Healthcare should not be regulated or medicated by big pharma, and it should not mean being fed processed (dead) food and GMOs by our corporate food companies.

No, true health reform is about clean living, eating nutrient-rich meals, being active, and taking responsibility for your life and its longevity. To change the culture of healthcare, there must be a change in the culture of doctors treating the public—a new breed of doctors focusing on what constitutes healthy patients. To reform healthcare, we must change what healthcare means.

There must be a new breed of doctor to bring that metaphoric change. Doctors practice what they teach by becoming healthier themselves. They focus on wellness rather than managed illness and sick care. There should be a focus on real nutrition, not drugs or the latest costly cosmetic procedure to fix the consequences of poor lifestyle and nutritional choices.

I believe society is in great need of an innovative new breed of doctors that use evidenced-based, natural, nutritional, restorative, and preventative care—doctors with a focus on lasting results, not temporary symptomatic results. A new breed addressing the true nature of health problems, not masking symptoms. Doctors who treat the cause and not the disease. Doctors focused on educating their patients to avoid becoming a medical nightmare.

This new breed of doctors can get the job done at huge savings to the patient and our economy. They can create change safely, effectively, and without the disabling or deadly (life-threatening side-effects) risks of over-medicating. Yes, the new breed can create a healthier world for us all to live in, rather than one with "accepted" protocols that don't focus on the patient's best interest at all.

Sick No More

It is time for a new approach to wellness, vitality, and longevity. If something is broken, it must be fixed, right? Well, we must first fix our expectations on vitality and longevity, rather than expecting illness as a part of life and the poor outcomes that go along with it. We must expect to prevent in most cases and treat for better outcomes in the few illnesses that may escape preventative measures. The pathway forward is to have knowledge. This way you are fighting the underlying causes, not the symptoms, as your sole focus.

Anyone taking acid reflux medication cannot call themselves healthy—the absence of symptoms does not equate to good health. Anyone taking cholesterol lowering drugs is not healthy, either. Someone regulating their blood pressure is sick, not well, regardless of what their readings are under medical management. Being regulated or medicated to control one's bloodwork not being in a state of optimal health is far from ideal. The new wave of cutting-edge doctors will use protocols that balance one's body chemistry instead, thus restoring health by treating the cause of dysfunction and disease.

We should not let ourselves down by surrendering to our body's decay!

Healthy vs. Fit

Health is a state in which all the components of the body are functioning properly. It is the absence of disease. Fit (fitness) is the ability to perform strenuous work or exercise. Notice fit and healthy are two different definitions. Is it possible to be one and not the other?

Fit & Unfit

Fit individuals are more likely to be healthier than unfit people. Since they are fit, fit people are seldom concerned with their weight. Even though they are fit, they cannot just relax. There are things they too can do to fight off the hands of time or their genetic profile. For instance, they should systemically detox often to improve health markers to match their fitness levels and dedication (i.e., avoid recreational and prescription drugs, blood pressure and cholesterol medication, SSRIs, and diet pills, etc.).

Can someone who regulates and medicates to obtain desired bloodwork panels really label themselves as fit and healthy? Few fit, healthy people struggle with health issues such as sleep apnea, diabetes, or blood pressure issues. Those who do may be fit, but obviously they are not what I consider healthy.

If you are not necessarily fit but also don't belong in the "healthy" category, you still have something to work with and time to work on what many have already lost, like healthy muscle. If you hold onto healthy muscle throughout your life by investing in a little extra exercise, that alone can make a huge difference in your health and life outcomes.

It is very difficult to obtain more muscle later in life once it is lost. Especially if you're not supplementing with branched-chain amino acids (BCAAs), which are not found in many foods. BCAAs are vital as we age, as they ensure protein utilization after assimilation. High-intensity exercises of short duration have proven to work best to maintain your accumulated quality of muscle.

Weight resistance is also a great way to keep up your muscle. You don't need to be a body builder, but you should at least be trying some program. The important thing is that we continue to build our strength by investing in our body. We need our muscles so that we can do things like lift our groceries and protect us from injuries. You may think it is silly to talk about lifting groceries, but as you age that will become more and more difficult if you don't invest in your muscles now.

In the end, it is important to decide what you like best within the area of keeping your body fit and trim. You will learn more on exercise later in the book, but the key is to start thinking about what you can do to support the body that supports you. It may just be that you like weight training and walking/running. It may be that you like swimming and yoga. I think variety in maintaining fitness is just as important as nutritional variety.

Fit for Life

The choice is yours as to whether you choose to take up staying fit now or wait for a more urgent occasion. The power to choose is yours, and yours alone. No one else holds the power to your health unless you choose to hand it over to them. Radiant health is yours if you so choose. The consequence of the alternative is also yours to bear if you don't.

Being Healthy

Being healthy and fit first demands our worthiness. We must know that we deserve a life where we thrive, not merely survive. We deserve a life worthy of the achievements that come from radiant health! Our investment in ourselves should not be seen as a sacrifice. Start early in becoming an active, productive agent in the outcome involving your health.

Don't delay, otherwise you will find yourself being reactive to disease and chronic health issues. We are creatures of habit, and so are our children. Therein lies the key to preventing bad health habits. It is not genetics that predisposes us to the health problems of our parents or surroundings. It is the repeating of their poor choices. The sooner we adopt positive habits, the sooner we will be able to pass them on to those we love: our friends and family. Examples speak louder than words.

Healthy/Fit in a Room

A healthy and fit person in a room draws so much attention and interest today. Just think about social media and how people show their perfect, filtered and altered pictures. Don't be deceived. Being healthy and fit is not about a look, it is about a feeling—feeling good, healthy, and energetic!

That said, there are numerous studies you can research about how attractive people get more advantages in life. Being healthy and fit is typically part of the attraction. For instance, when you think about the sex symbols on TV, they appear to be healthy and fit, right? If you are not worried about being a sex symbol on TV, you should still do your research. For instance, try taking an in-depth look at the following studies:

- A published study in the *Journal of Labor Research* found that physically fit people can earn more money and are more likely to be employed, promoted, and have higher job satisfaction.[11]
- A published study in the *Journal of Personality and Social Psychology* found that physically fit people are perceived as more attractive. This can lead to more favorable treatment, including more social opportunities.[12]
- A published study in the *International Journal of Obesity* found that individuals who are obese are less likely to be hired and more likely to be passed over for promotions. The data suggests that maintaining a healthy weight could lead to more workplace opportunities.[13]
- A published study in the journal *Frontiers in Psychology* found individuals who are physically fit typically have better cognitive function. This includes things like better memory and attention spans, which can lead to more opportunities in academics and professionally.[14]

Don't kill the messenger if you don't like what you read above. I want to give you every motivation to invest more in yourself so you can improve your life beyond your looks and physical body. You can have more opportunities in all aspects of your life, including your employment, social interactions, cognitive performance, and more. Now, are you motivated?

---

[11] Lechner, M. D., & Franck, E. (2016). The earnings and employment benefits of physical activity: Evidence from the Canadian National Population Health Survey. Journal of Labor Research, 37(2), 181-209.

[12] Jackson, L. A., Hunter, J. E., & Hodge, C. N. (1995). Physical attractiveness and intellectual competence: A meta-analytic review. Journal of Personality and Social Psychology, 68(4), 768-781.

[13] Puhl, R. M., & Heuer, C. A. (2009). The stigma of obesity: A review and update. Obesity, 17(5), 941-964.

[14] Ludyga, S., Gerber, M., & Brand, S. (2016). Association between cardiorespiratory fitness and cognitive function in healthy men and women: A cross-sectional study. Frontiers in Psychology, 7, 1742.

It is alarming when the "norm" becomes an exception. Even 50 years ago, when a 200-lb. man walked in a room, he was considered a large man. Today, people *over* 200 lb. are everywhere—both male and female. Big is in! Fit is fading, and the new normal is unnatural (being unfit). We've got to get our minds out of the fat-free '70s if we want to rid ourselves of the fat butts everyone started acquiring in the '80s and beyond. There are answers, and yes, you can do it! You can be fit, trim, strong, and healthy!

Fundamentals That Develop a Healthy and Fit Life

Every level of your health is directly impacted by what you eat. If it were all about calories, food would be simple. Food is not just for energy or calories, it's a source of information that gives instructions to your body to either upgrade or downgrade your biological system with every bite. Food regulates not only your genes, but also hormones (like insulin, estrogens, testosterone, thyroid, and cortisol). It alters our brain chemistry, making us happy or depressed. It can also sadly even lead to addictive patterns. Food can either create or prevent inflammatory conditions (like joint pain, IBS, dermatitis, ADD/ADHD, and most autoimmune disorders) and enhance or destroy your immune system.

The key is to personalize your diet and nutritional needs. You set your plan to whatever fits your needs. A few examples are below. Eat to:

- Build bones
- Balance your hormones
- Build muscle
- Lose or gain weight
- Fix your gut
- Boost your immunity
- Improve heart health
- Gain energy
- Reduce fat
- Look good in jeans or a bikini
- FOR ANY REASON!!!

WHAT CAN I DO?

When you are eating something, ask yourself if you are fine with it as part of your long-term goals. If not, don't eat it. Instead, seek out a better-quality substitute to meet your goals.

Food Groups: My personal recommendations:

- Proteins @ 40% (animal sources are best)
- Carbohydrates @ 20% (eat the rainbow!)
- Fats @ 40% (eat with every meal)

Protein:

Life Unfolds with Protein

"Protein is the living, respiring substance that needs to be fueled and supplied with oxygen to sustain combustion and provide energy for the unique material that is life itself. Regulating every function in the body."
Jen Moller, M.D.

The best source for building muscle is eating muscle. Animal proteins are the best choice. Plant proteins are alright, but the quality is lower, and they contain significantly less BCAAs, which are necessary for optimal strength and vitality.

- Examples: Grass-fed animals or wild meats, wild fish, organic eggs, liver, venison, beef, organic chicken, duck, etc.
- Fish: Wild fish is best. Avoid farmed fish—they contain GMOs and are high in proinflammatory omega-6 fatty acids (as opposed to wild fish, which are high in anti-inflammatory omega-3 fatty acids).
- Fish & Seafood
  - Benefits: High in omega-3 essential fatty acids, pro-anti-inflammatory, low glycemic index
  - (Bake, broil, or grill ... but avoid frying)

○ Wild caught salmon (not farm raised), tuna, snapper, sea bass, tilapia, flounder, grouper, herring, sardine, trout, shrimp, and lobster

Carbohydrates:

Non-starchy veggies are the gold standard. Veggies, such as those from the cruciferous family, are best. Kale, broccoli, Brussels sprouts, cauliflower, collard greens, or spinach should cover 2/3 of your plate each day. These also happen to be what is known as estrogen 2-16 regulators, which are powerful cancer suppressors, due in part to their high methyl group donors.

A healthy, lean female body is made up of 55 percent water, 16 percent protein, 22 percent fat, 6 percent minerals, and just 1 percent carbohydrates. The problem is that most of our western processed diets are composed of 50-60 percent carbohydrates (like starches and sugars). The body can literally survive and thrive without any carbohydrate consumption.

- Grains and Pasta:
    - ○ Benefits: None
    - ○ Neutral: Quinoa, organic brown rice/wild rice, barley, rye flour, kasha, spelt flour
    - ○ Breads: Ezekiel, Essene, 100% Rye

- Cereals
    - ○ Benefits: None
    - ○ Neutral: Kasha, amaranth, barley, spelt, buckwheat, rice broth

Fats:

Fat is the most misunderstood food group. I know this is going to sound crazy out there to many, but you should try to have a serving of fat with every meal. In fact, certain fats are essential to your life, which cannot be said about carbohydrates.

Polyunsaturated fats are best—like fish oils, flaxseed, or grass-fed animals. They are all loaded with omega-3s and some omega-6s, which are the building blocks of life. Monosaturated fats like olive oils, avocados, nuts, etc. also improve insulin sensitivity by balancing blood sugar.

Coconut oil has really taken on excellent press as of late. It is a medium-chain triglyceride, loved by the body's mitochondria, which is the workhorse of the cell. It is great for pre-workout energy (I suggest a tablespoon in liquid form or spoon fed, whatever you prefer) and has been documented to improve brain function and energy.

Our bodies can't make these fats; therefore, they must be consumed. In a perfect world, our diets would be one part omega-3 fatty acid to one to two parts omega-6 fatty acid. Unfortunately, the American diet is one part omega-3 fatty acid to 25 or greater part omega-6 fatty acid, which ultimately leads us to chronic inflammation issues including the so-called metabolic syndrome, syndrome X, obesity, type II diabetes, cardiovascular disease, joint pains, and more.

Don't fear fat. We don't live in the '70s anymore. Eat quality fats with every meal. Fats don't make you fat unless you eat them with starches or sugars. Fats do not raise insulin levels. If you don't raise insulin levels, you don't accumulate fat. That is physiology 101. The few exceptions are trans-fats, which you should avoid at all costs. Your body takes weeks to break down trans-fats, and they can lead to heart disease.

Beans & Legumes
- Benefits: Black-eye peas, pinto beans
- Neutral: Black beans, green beans, northern beans, lima beans, string beans, white beans, red beans, and garbanzo beans

Dairy
- Benefits: None
- Neutral: (Natural/real) butter, feta, goat cheese, mozzarella, casein, almond milk, goat milk, rice milk, and blue cheese

*If cow dairy milk is a must, stay organic!

Vegetables
- Benefits: Loaded with antioxidants, low glycemic levels, good source of fiber, many contain methyl groups
- Asparagus, Broccoli, Brussels sprouts, cabbage, carrots, cauliflower, kale, mushrooms, onion, parsley, pumpkin, scallion, snow peas, squash, sweet potato, tomato, watercress

*Protect your flavonoids. Eat raw or crisp, steamed is best, and bake if you must—NEVER microwave!

Drinks
- Benefits: Hydration, detoxification, purification
- Filtered water, green tea, kukicha/bancha haiku, wine, and glacier water/deuterium depleted water (DDW)

*NO tap water, and NO sodas!

Nuts
- Benefits: Great source of healthy fats, satisfies hunger cravings
- Pecans, almonds, walnuts, cashews, and Brazil nuts

Soups
- Benefits: Great alternative to regular vegetable consumption
- Miso soup, seaweed soup, ginger soup, and lentil soup

Seasonings
- Benefits: Many medicinal purposes, great flavor additive
- Turmeric, onions, garlic, herbs, pepper (try varieties*), sea salt, lemon juice, and real butter (NO margarine*)

Other food items
- Balsamic or wine vinegar, pickles/brine, sauerkraut, mayonnaise, mustard, and Italian olive salad

The Sweets

- <u>Sweeteners</u>:
  - ○ Benefits: None
  - ○ Raw honey, Stevia, and maple syrup (real)

- <u>Sugars</u>:
  - ○ Treat sugar like a recreational drug
  - ○ The dose makes the difference ... an occasional sweet treat is harmless

Flour is even worse than sugar for the body, and bread is the absolute worst. We have hundreds of genes protecting us from starvation, but few protecting us from abundance and overconsumption. Lepton is a hormone that regulates when we are sated with our caloric intake per meal. Due to increased insulin dysregulation, this hormone loses its ability to regulate the body's feeling of when hunger is satisfied.

We live in a sea of sugar causing our biology, especially our hormones (brain chemistry and immune systems), to go haywire in the form of autoimmune disorders, increased cravings, fat storage, slowed metabolism, and an epidemic of obesity, cardiovascular disease, diabetes, cancer, and dementia. It all comes down to a global insulin resistance problem. In fact, one in two Americans (and one in every four teenagers) are prediabetic and overweight according to a CDC study published in *JAMA Pediatrics*. Why are such obesity ridden diseases plaguing our society today? It is sugars and starch, not fat, that is killing us all.

Once or twice a year, a sugar detox can help reset your body. All you need is a 10-day reset (example: Dr. Jones' Phase 1 Diet Plan). This is not a quick fix or a deprivation diet. It is a system that works by using real whole foods and the right nutrients to reset your system and support healthy blood sugar. However, if you are overweight, have type II diabetes, or are prediabetic, a longer-term reset may be needed to repair your metabolism.

A healthy relationship with sugar is when you do not crave it or need it every day. A few categories of sugar that I recommend cutting out completely are:

- High-fructose corn syrup
- Sugar alcohols
- All fake sugars and sugar substitutes (Stevia is a good substitute; Splenda is not)
- Avoid sweets with meals, as this increases AGEs

*For more information on Dr. Jones' Phase I Diet plan for Balancing Body Chemistry, visit www.DrJoeyJones.com.

Things to Avoid

- Nitrates
- Breads
- Fried foods
- Table salt (use sea salt)
- Preservatives
- Sodas
- MSG
- Margarine (use real butter)
- High-fructose corn syrup
- ALL high glycemics

Water

Deuterium depleted water (DDW) is the best. DDW inhibits cell proliferation, meaning it has potential as an adjunct to anti-tumor therapy. Deuterium in water interferes with mitochondria function, thus slowing down energy production and increasing the promotion of free radicals. Deuterium water is more commonly known as *heavy water*. The healthiest form of DDW is typically spring water—mountain and glacial springs are superior.

For water, I recommend consumption of at least 1 oz. per 2 lbs. of body weight; an example would be a 160 lb. person consuming 80 oz. of water per day. Note, I said *water*, not *fluids*. You will preferably consume glacier spring water, if you can. Heavy water, which is most of the unfiltered water used in homes in city municipalities, contains high levels of fluoride, chlorine, and bromine, all of which are well known toxins.

Don't fear—there are so many ways you can put more water in your diet that can be fun. You can incorporate water into soups, smoothies, popsicles with fruit, and so on!

Weight Loss Guaranteed with the Side Effect of Radiant Health

In my opinion, there is no debate as to what the perfect human diet is. The answer, as usual, can be found in simplicity. It is the very diet that got us through the last hundreds of thousands of years. There is really no debate over portions of carbohydrates vs. fats or proteins. Like I said, this diet has got us through since the beginning of mankind: a protein-based diet. Protein is the single most important element to survival, period. For the nay-sayers, I recommend the must-see documentary *The Perfect Human Diet*, directed and produced by C.J. Hunt.

Life Unfolds with Protein

"Protein is the living, respiring substance that needs to be fueled and supplied with oxygen to sustain combustion and provide energy for the unique material that is like itself, regulating every function in the body."
Jen Moller, M.D.

Protein is the substance that all biochemical and physiological activity in life relies on. The normal condition of a living organism is a balance between anabolic (protein building) and catabolic (protein destroying) processes.

As far as weight loss is concerned, keep it simple. No need to dive deep into the physiological goings on to get leaner and healthier. Fat accumulation (growth) is caused by a hormone 99% of the time.

Just as we grow taller through hormones, we also grow heavier and fatter through the release of the hormone insulin. Release as little insulin as possible when you eat, and you will not gain weight from fat, period. Notice that I'm not even mentioning exercise, low-calorie starvation diets, calorie counting, or point systems.

It's simple. Release as little of the hormone insulin from the pancreas during meals to achieve weight loss. Let's break down some common food types and see if they affect insulin release.

Food	Glycemic Index/ Glucose Effect	Insulin Released
○ Eggs	Low	Next to none
○ Porkchops/bacon	Low	Next to none
○ Chicken	Low	Next to none
○ Salad greens	Low	Minimum
○ Red meats	Low	Next to none
○ Bread	High	Large
○ Fruits	Medium	Moderate
○ Nuts	Low	Very little
○ Dairy	Medium	Moderate
○ Fish	Low	Next to none

You can probably guess by now that I'm not a big fan of diets or eating habits that use grains and particular breads, pastas, etc. in their protocols. The major concern here is the high glycemic and pro-inflammatory effects of glutens found in these food groups. I find many patients suffering with weight problems also suffer with inflammatory health conditions as well, including almost all autoimmune disorders and digestive problems like IBS, diabetes, lupus, arthritis, fibromyalgia, depression, anxiety, multiple sclerosis, and more. These are all conditions that grains and gluten can impact.

Calorie counting and point system diets fail to take into consideration the inflammatory side effects and allergic reactions that are major complications associated with grains (especially when trying to maintain and sustain weight loss). These side-effects are not found in protein and fat-based diets or even diets utilizing low glycemic vegetables for carbohydrate consumption.

- Key Points:
  - ➢ No exercises needed
  - ➢ Simply put your pancreas down for a nap
  - ➢ Wake it up slowly (as you would want to be awakened)

- The beauty lies in the side effects:
  - ➢ Reversing type II diabetes
  - ➢ Bringing most blood pressure issues under control
  - ➢ Eliminate acid reflux
  - ➢ Reduce systemic (whole body) inflammation
  - ➢ Improve overall blood work
  - ➢ Possible reversal of sleep apnea issues
  - ➢ RADIANT HEALTH!

For more information and individualized programs on this subject, go to www.DrJoeyJones.com.

The Enemy… CARBOHYDRATES (i.e., Refined Sugars and White Flour)

There are many, many foods in the typical American diet today that are slowly killing us, including any foods with refined sugars and white flour, both of which are *vastly* overconsumed.

Some things to consider before you put anything else in your mouth:

- Processed and high glycemic carbohydrates stop the body from producing the muscle-building and anti-aging growth hormone glucagon.

- Just two sodas of any kind (diet or regular) a day can change the body from fat burning into fat gaining mode.
- Humans don't require any processed carbs and only need very few natural carbs. One of the most common causes of not losing body fat is essential fatty acids deficiency and mineral deficiency. This drives us to consume too many processed carbs and results in elevated blood glucose levels, thus releasing insulin into circulation.
- Eat a diet used to fatten a cow (grain and corn) and you will achieve the same.
- Carbohydrates (sugars) don't contribute directly to anything except excess body fat through elevated insulin secretions.
- Processed carbs (sodas, school lunches, etc.) plague our children with sugar highs and sugar lows all day long. These highs and lows lead to a lack of attention and focus, making learning difficult. An example of this is the epidemic proportions of ADD and ADHD plaguing our youth. EFA (essential fatty acids) help eliminate cravings for processed carbs, thus helping reduce or even eliminate these symptoms.

Proteins and fats should be balanced with carbohydrates. Here lies the problem most of us are confused about. What constitutes a carbohydrate? Most of us think of pasta, sweets, and potatoes. *THINK fruits and vegetables instead!

Favorable and Unfavorable Carbohydrates

Definition of (a) favorable or (b) unfavorable is based on the concept of the glycemic load.

> (A.) *Favorable carbohydrates* have a low capacity to stimulate insulin (low glycemic load). Favorable carbs = low effect on insulin

Examples:
1. Most vegetables
2. Most fruits (except bananas and raisins)
3. Select grains (like oatmeal)

(B.) *Unfavorable carbohydrates* are just the opposite, as they stimulate high levels of insulin (high glycemic index). Unfavorable carbs = greater effect on insulin

Examples:
1. Grains and starches (pastas, breads, cereal, potatoes, and carrots)
2. Select fruits (bananas, raisins)

We Need to Fall in Love with Protein

Every meal must have protein for these reasons:

1. The body needs to replace the protein that is lost from the body daily.
2. Protein stimulates the release of the hormone glucagon. This hormone tells your body to release stored carbohydrates from the liver to maintain adequate blood sugar levels for the brain.
3. Glucagon acts as a brake for secreted excess insulin. So, if your glucagon level increases, insulin levels decrease.

Fat Facts

It takes fat to burn fat. Here again, there are good fats and bad fats.

Good fats fall into two categories:

* Monounsaturated
* Long-chain-omega-3 fats (polyunsaturated fats)

Monounsaturated fats come from olive oil, select nuts, avocados, etc. Long chain-omega-3 fats come from fish, fish oil, flaxseed, and grass-fed meats.

You want to restrict **bad fats** from your diets!

Bad fats include:

- Saturated fats
- Arachidonic acid
- Trans fats

Saturated fats are found in fatty cuts of red meat and high-fat dairy products. Trans fats are artificial fats created by the food industry and are in virtually all processed foods.

Example: "partially hydrogenated vegetable oils"

Note: *Avoid trans fats at all costs!

Arachidonic acid: Found primarily in fatty red meats, organ meats, and egg yolks. The higher your insulin levels, the more your body is stimulated to make increased levels of arachidonic acid. Serum AA/EPA—Ideal=1.5. Most Americans @ 11. Danger zone >10. Chronic disease >15.

Essential Fatty Acids (EFAs)

Lastly, I want to elaborate on the most important fats of all. EFAs are essential for survival, healthy growth, and anti-aging.

Forget the opinions of those who have been conditioned to believe health, appearance, and performance can be improved by avoiding fats.

Two critical EFAs are alpha-linolenic (omega-3) and alpha-linoleic (omega-6) fatty acids. They are lipotropic (promote the transportation and utilization of fats and help prevent accumulation of fats in the liver) and anabolic (which is key to the constructive phase of metabolism; for example, muscle building agents). Thus, they help to increase muscle and decrease fat.

These types of fats also relieve pain and help improve mood, energy, healing, memory, vision, and joint repair. They are especially useful when on low-carb diets because they encourage the body to use available fats for energy.

EFAs: Basically, these help your body become more of a fat burning machine ... in other words, they dig into your body fat storage to supply your metabolic demands.

Once you get control of your diet, the effects will be almost instantaneous for many. Others may experience more impacts over time as their body heals itself. Another key to jumpstarting your health is fasting.

Intermediate/Intermittent Fasting

While intermittent fasting, it is best to have the first meal of the day after 10 a.m. and the last meal completed by 6 p.m. This supports the elimination cycle of the body, which takes place between 4 a.m. and noon, thus increasing the possibility of multiple bowel movements during this period. Listen to your body and know your health conditions before starting a fasting schedule. Some people may require a protein or fat snack during the night to balance blood sugar drops during early fasting stages.

Fasting has so many beneficial impacts, including:

- Increased vitality
- Increased longevity
- Improved cognitive function
- Improved overall mood
- Aided weight loss

Fasting is not a diet. We are even told of the benefits of fasting in the Bible. So, consider all your options when you think about how to best reach your health goals, including going on a spiritual fast with a purpose in mind.

Keep in mind there are several famous verses in the Bible that mention fasting. Here are a few of them:

> *"Is not this the kind of fasting I have chosen: to loose*
> *the chains of injustice and untie the cords of the yoke,*
> *to set the oppressed free and break every yoke?"*
> Isaiah 58:6 (NIV)

> *"While they were worshiping the Lord and fasting,*
> *the Holy Spirit said, 'Set apart for me Barnabas*
> *and Saul for the work to which I have called them.'*
> *So after they had fasted and prayed, they placed*
> *their hands on them and sent them off."*
> Acts 13:2-3 (NIV)

Whatever your reason for fasting, I want to give you the basics to motivate you to consider it in your overall health plan. For instance, survival genes increase their overall function when fasting. They become activated on low caloric intakes. One such example is the use of starvation diets in the suppression treatment of cancers.

When snacking during intermediate fasting, try to snack on foods high in fat and as close to the end of your last meal as possible to avoid hunger surges. Examples of snacks include nuts—pecans are best because of their fat to protein ratio (7/1). Keep in mind that every food you consume triggers an insulin reaction. Proteins and fats trigger the least, whereas carbohydrates secrete the highest reaction. So, the less often you eat, the less often insulin is released.

Your first meal of the day (say between 10 a.m. and noon) should be higher in protein and fats with the largest calorie content. Your next meal (3-4 hours later) preferably should contain approximately 8 oz. veggies and salad (consumed with olive oil and vinegar, nuts, seeds, etc.) as this helps to balance blood sugar and has high anti-diabetic effects. Also, spices like turmeric are anti-inflammatory.

Again, the best time to snack with high-fat foods is at the end of a meal, as it helps reduce hunger cravings later. The best time for snacking overall is between the first and second meal, as it helps increase total fasting times. If a third meal is necessary, try to eat a mix of low-calorie protein, fat, and veggies with a fat snack soon after if needed.

Side effects are weight loss, improved energy and mood, and cognitive sharpness. Expect some muscle loss due to decreased protein consumption, which is typically associated with consuming fewer meals.

Dr. J's Perfect Bite

If you are looking for what I consider the simple path to freedom by enhancing your health, try out meals like these with intermittent fasting:

#1.
1 boiled egg
2 slices of bacon or sausage links/patties
1 small avocado
4-6 Kalamata olives
½ oz. or so feta cheese
Celtic or Himalaya salt
Ground pepper
Cover in olive oil/dressing

#2.
6 ounces arugula or favorite greens
1-2 tbsp pecans or walnuts
½-1 oz. feta or parmesan cheese
¼ cup strawberries/blueberries
Olive oil and vinegar
½ of a lemon's juice
4 oz. protein: salmon, chicken, red meat, tuna, etc.
*Omit fruits if the purpose of your meals is weight loss

*If the primary purpose of your meals is moderate weight loss, add a protein-only meal before and after examples #1 and #2 along with mineral supplementation.

The Skinny on Being Fit for Life

If you get nothing else from this chapter, remember this: If you significantly restrict or eliminate starchy carbs and sugars while eliminating glutens from your diet, keep your protein consumption adequate (around 40-80 grams per day) and eat as much good fats as necessary to satisfy your appetite. If you can pull that off, your overall health and well-being will improve remarkably, you'll live longer, and you will age more gracefully. And that's all without expensive fad diets, diabetic medications, supplements, or surgeries. **Put simply**: The less carbohydrates you consume, the healthier you will be, and the longer you are likely to live. Why? Because less carbs = less insulin secreted = a longer life.

Cleanse, Detoxification, & Fortification

In addition to fasting, there are other things that you can do to reboot your health, including a cleanse, detox, and fortification. This is one of my favorite tools in my toolbox to help my clients achieve more positive outcomes in their lives.

Let's Talk Detoxification:

Cleansing (or detoxification) has to do with reducing the burden of infection and toxicity in the body. It is the event of reducing the metabolic load placed upon the body by metabolic waste byproduct (such as food toxins, heavy metals, and poisons like prescription medications, high-fructose corn syrup, fluoride, chlorine, etc.), thus causing the body to function at a more exhausting rate.

   Although the initial cleanse/detox is considered a first step and involves dealing with many years' worth of acquired neglect and stored up contaminants, the initial release is often more dramatic and potent.

However, cleansing is never actually finished because life itself is a toxic endeavor requiring constant micro-cleansing. The results are a dramatic reduction in allergic complexes throughout the body, as they have been wreaking much havoc on our immune systems.

Simple undetected chronic food allergies, like wheat or dairy, occupy so much activity in our immune systems that once these allergens are removed the immune system is free to perform the responsibilities that were neglected when it was stressed out and overburdened.

After Detox, You Must Fortify:

Generally, nutrients are responsible for initiating repair and fortification. There are basically two metabolic pathways at work in our bodies: anabolism (to build up), and catabolism (to break down). Anabolism is responsible for growth and repair, whereas catabolism (catabolic) is responsible for breakdown and recycling. The balance between these two activities determines whether you are growing and thriving or shrinking and degenerating.

The process of fortification is partially under the function of the hormonal system (such as the anabolic hormone testosterone or the catabolic hormone cortisone, in addition to others). Suppling the body with adequate nutrient materials such as proteins, minerals, and essential fatty acids encourages hormonal balance and the necessary growth factors for tissue repair and improving the metabolic process.

Getting a hold on one's stress early in life—say, during the ages of 20 and 40—will have a greater influence over the rate of one's declining health. This is what I call the "disease years" when symptoms start to present themselves. This declining health tends to be in proportion to the degree of stimulation endured by glandular structures, such as adrenal, thyroid, and pituitary, and the resulting damage placed upon our fortification process.

THE SCIENCE OF NATURAL HYGIENE

Natural hygiene recognizes that the human body is an organism that is constantly striving for wellness. "Natural hygiene" implies a cleanliness of the body that is achieved through natural, non-contrived means. The underlying basis is that the body is self-cleansing, self-healing, and self-maintaining. We experience problems of ill health (i.e., excess weight, pain, and stress) only when we break the natural laws of life.

The science of natural hygiene revolves around the following topics:

- Understanding the body's natural hygiene digestive cycles
- Correct consumption of food groups
- The concept of high-water/content food
- Correct food combining

THE BODY'S NATURAL DIGESTIVE CYCLES

The human body's digestive system goes through three eight-hour cycles every day:

APPROPRIATION: NOON - 8 P.M. (eating & digesting)
ASSIMILATION: 8 P.M. - 4 A.M. (absorption & use)
ELIMINATION: 4 A.M. - NOON (excretion of waste)

APPROPRIATION - (Noon - 8 p.m.) Our bodies crave nourishment during the appropriation period. Most Americans begin this cycle too early and therefore cancel the elimination phase. The most important rule during appropriation is to eat only when your body is hungry.

Nighttime is not a good time for appropriation (eating & digesting) because digestion works best when assisted by gravity and functions very poorly at horizontal angles (lying down). If you leave three hours between your last meal and when you go to bed, your food has left your stomach and is well on its way through the alimentary tract. At this point, it is extracting nutrients in the assimilation phase.

ASSIMILATION - (8 p.m. - 4 a.m.) Assimilation occurs mostly at night and ideally must begin on time. Assimilation at night makes sense because the body is resting the digestive system and is regulated by the parasympathetic nervous system, which is ready to kick into gear without interruption. During assimilation, the body extracts nutrients in our intestine, which are 12 times the length of our intestinal cavity and designed to keep dietary foods in their clutches until all nutrients are withdrawn.

ELIMINATION - (4 a.m. - noon) Elimination is simply the removal of waste matter from the body. Your body has sorted through food it has processed and rejected food debris that cannot be absorbed. The body also eliminates toxins that accumulate in the body via the underarm, the bowel, urine, glands behind the knees, and from the nose, mouth, ears, and skin.

Elimination is the most thwarted digestive cycle of the three. This abuse has led to chronic constipation, obesity, and catastrophic ill health in our society. The elimination cycle is almost always sabotaged by us unwittingly eating a poor breakfast, which prevents the body from executing its essential daily function of removing waste from the body. The result of such behavior is that we consume three to four meals a day with one or zero bowl movements. Finally, we look at ourselves in the mirror one day, in horror, and exclaim, "Good grief, I look like a beached whale!"

If that's how you feel, it's time to unplug yourself, Einstein, and get rid of the whale!

Hot/Sluggish Gallbladder

<u>Signs and Symptoms</u>:

1. Light colored stools
2. Mid/upper back pain (around shoulder blades, sometimes with acute painful exacerbation in early morning hours)
3. Sensitivity to fatty foods (i.e., indigestion, distressed stomach, loss of appetite, sudden need to eliminate)

<u>Cause</u>:
Usually associated with a failure in the mechanism of bile flow due to many causes. Many patients formally considered as operable may be restored to asymptomatic basis with proper therapy early. Response where stones are present largely depends on the type of stones.

<u>Specific Treatment Protocol</u>:
1. Betaine Therapy: Greatest source found in young beet leave products containing B vitamin factors, which help lower the viscosity of bile.
2. Choline: B vitamin derivative involved in fat metabolism and digestion; supports the action of bile salts in emulsifying fats.
3. Betaine Hydrochloride: Improves gastric secretion and protein digestion, both of which are very important in all gallbladder problems.
4. Disodium Phosphate: Liver and gallbladder stimulant. Stimulates bile flow. This is for when stones are present in the gallbladder.

Hold on to your gallbladder at all costs. It has major functions in your biliary digestion and assimilation systems. A plethora of possible health complications lay in store once it is removed.

So You Want to Tame Your Telomeres and Slow Down the Biological Merry-Go-Round?

How We Age:

The definition of ideology (reason) is the science of ideas or thought or a philosophy. There can be found a great deal of clinical information and theories to the proximate cause of aging (i.e, senescence). And there is also a plethora of theories as to why we die, most of which defy any reputable testing. I'll save my opinion for a latter print though. Sadly, most of the early research on how and why we age has been put on a shelf over the past 50-plus years in favor of the highly lucrative science of treating the symptoms of senescence—better known as Geriatric Medicine.

One theory that is showing rapid advanced scientific interest, including my own, is that of the biological molecular effects of cellular death. The biology of cellular death is believed to be the primary index of senescence. Literature points to proteins that accumulate in the blood, tissue fluids, and connective tissues of mammals as age increases. These accumulations tend to store up in the body.

Normally, certain elimination factors (i.e., sex hormones, thyroid, adrenals, etc.) remove the proteins from the connective tissue storehouse and transfer them into the tissue fluids or blood, where they are then utilized for tissue repair or excreted from the organism. As age increases, the organs responsible for elimination (i.e., gonads, thymus, and thyroid) and excretion (liver, spleen, blood, kidneys, etc.) progressively regress, throwing the whole elimination cycle out of balance. Thus, the primary cause of senescence can be linked to a progressive protein build-up over time.

A direct consequence of an impaired protein elimination system is the resulting gradual accumulation of toxic (waste) byproducts. These accumulations lower cell potential by lowering cellular PH and preventing mitosis, which in turn decreases cellular vitality and telomere length and eventually leads to death of the organism. Promoters of telomere shortening and expenditure of the metabolic cycle (i.e., aging and senescence) include cellular protein build-up, increased cortisol levels (stress), increased insulin levels (diabetes), decreased sex hormones, and decreased CoQ10 levels, to name just a few. To see a more in-depth list, visit www.DrJoeyJones.com.

To increase cellular vitality and longevity, the body must involve these key players in intra and extra-cellular reactions necessary to maximize cellular regeneration and repair. A few key players include vitamin B complex (an important adjunct to slowing the progression of most all degenerative and debilitating diseases), chlorophyll (increases platelet counts, which are concerned with the elimination of toxic protein debris that accumulate in tissue fluids), CoQ10 (increases cellular oxidation, and vital for energy production), lecithin (key component in phospholipid formation, necessary for protein debris elimination, and a natural antagonist to cholesterol), methyl groups (such as cruciferous vegetables, which are critical in the metabolic cycle of protein sheathing and elimination), and RNA (the growth promoter when added to tissue, associated with protein synthesis and cell division).

Here's a hypothesis: Life span is determined by some key organ or master gland that is "wound up like an intrinsic clock," perhaps set at around the eighth decade in biological years and that gradually runs down during the metabolic activities associated with the life cycle. Protein metabolism strongly suggests it is the master gland (anterior pituitary) whose control of the life cycle is in turn determined (perhaps by heredity features). Its medium of determination of the life cycle may revolve around its control over the system of elimination of proteins and other cellular waste byproducts. Particularly concerning is its relationship with the maintenance of the immune system.

A great example here is natural calorie reduction in the elderly as they age. By reducing the amount of excess metabolic energy needed for digestion, more metabolic cellular energy reserves can be used in cellular repair and protein debris elimination. Thus, the reduction of energy expenditure slows down the "unwinding" of one's "pre-wound metabolic clock." This ultimately slows one's metabolism with age and improves cellular and telomere longevity (i.e., their lifespan).

TO YOUR HEALTH

Hippocrates, who has been called the father of modern medicine, said, "First do no harm to the body." We need to accept that our current healthcare system is infested with problems and is most definitely doing our bodies harm.

Society is acknowledging this and making rapid changes. Over the last 20 years, alternative wellness-based health care has surpassed traditional sickness-based health care in total patient expenditure. Society is showing it wants a new healthcare system—one that takes nutrition and prevention of disease into consideration. Most doctors are not trained in nutrition because the institutions they receive their education from see nutrition and associated products as useless commercially.

So, their recommendations on what is best for your health are based on flawed assumptions to begin with, namely that drugs, surgical procedures, and cutting-edge medical techniques rather than nutrition are the cures for the ills of mankind. Doctors were taught this in institutions funded by drug companies.

Detoxification is, by its very nature, a preventive ethic, and so not normally appreciated by doctors not trained in prevention procedures. Prevention, it is often said, is the best cure.

Metabolic diseases are diseases that are related to our utilization of food. Approximately 90-95% of all diseases and health problems that are killing us today tend to be metabolic, toxin, or healthcare related in origin.

Metabolic diseases cannot be solved by anything other than the missing metabolic preventive, which is always a nutritional factor. In case you have not figured it out by now, that means that drugs foreign to the biological experience of the human body will never cure a metabolic disease. And what is currently being used by medical establishments to halt metabolic diseases? YOU GUESSED IT! DRUGS!

Changes are difficult for most human beings. How many times have you come across a friend, loved one, or even a physician who just does not see things the way you do? They do not see a problem or will not admit there is a problem, and so they remain unmoved by your passionate desires for change.

This makes me think of the quote from Max Planck, the Nobel Prize-winning German physicist: "A new scientific truth does not triumph by convincing its opponents and making them see the light, but rather because its opponents die, and a new generation grows up that is familiar with it." Which generation are you?

Your Reflection Corner

Chapter 6: What Can I Do?

Start Today

What better way is there to achieve good health than through a physically and mentally active lifestyle? Many of us believe health is something that belongs to the young and is taken from us as we age. The presence of a healthy person radiates energy, enthusiasm, putting a smile on one's face, and causing heads to turn.

As a society, we tend to regard physical health and vitality as something reserved for the young, and thus we place little emphasis on trying to maintain it and preserve it as we age. Then we panic at the first sign of declining health, energy, or physical appearance. We grasp at miracle cures, super diets, stimulants, relaxants, special tonics, and potions in hopes of preserving our youthful health and vitality.

Your healthy body is a gift from nature with a lifetime warranty. That body includes an all-too-often overlooked disclaimer: Use it without abusing it, or you will lose it.

Men and women, young and old, continue to enjoy pain-free, healthy, and active lifestyles with exercise, proper nutrition, and regular chiropractic care.

People not only say they feel better following chiropractic care, but they also often say they feel healthier, stronger, and more vibrant. They have a greater comprehension of the way their body functions and thus they understand the role chiropractic care, exercise, and proper nutrition play in the process of achieving superlative health. Through increased physical capabilities, a stronger mind, and improved health, you'll ultimately reach the threshold of optimal health. An active lifestyle is common for these people and a constant reminder of the impact it has on both our bodies and minds.

The natural beauty and the effortlessness we maintain in our youth becomes so transient and fragile in later years. Our natural ability to recover quickly from life's stresses and traumas in our youth diminishes as we age. We must change our health care philosophy to that of a more complex. preventive approach to survive as we venture into middle age. We are often unprepared for the processes that take us beyond the boundaries of optimal physical health. There are no easy-to-follow guidelines, magic diets, or secret remedies that lead us into middle age and beyond. Modern health care is finally beginning to place its interest in prevention and education of diseases and dysfunctional injuries, therefore helping to lead us into our healthier and more active so-called "golden years." The effort of chiropractic preventive or maintenance care with proper nutrition and exercise can create such an avenue for active lifestyles to come shining through.

Aging is a process that evolves for all of us as we travel down the road of life. It doesn't have to lead to a future of declining health or loss of the joys associated with an active lifestyle.

I personally believe a healthy body is one of life's greatest gifts. What we choose to do with it—use it, abuse it, or lose it—is determined to its greatest degree by us.

A balance of chiropractic care, exercise, and proper nutrition has kept me and millions of others in better shape physically, emotionally, and mentally through life's roller-coaster ride.

Life should continue to be as exciting and fulfilling from middle age through the golden years as it was in your youth.

Many practitioners today are dedicating themselves to the same approach of empowering the benefits of exercise and education for optimal health. This is a lifestyle many of us should practice and preach.

Some patients claim they don't have time to prepare a healthy diet or exercise even for 30 minutes two to three times a week. My sincere reply is, "You don't have time not to!"

Whatever your age, vitality comes with activity. So, get on with it and put that fear of aging behind you! Above all, doing so will lend a new quality to one of your most precious possessions—your health.

Today is the best day to start, as tomorrow new challenges and obstacles will be there to create new excuses for why you cannot create change in your life. To begin, ask yourself a few questions to determine where you should start.

If today was your last day, would you feel good about how you spent your time?

- What did you do today? Relive your day ... did you spend the time wisely?
- How did you feel today? Did you feel like you were really living or just surviving?
- Did you live with intensity to make your life and moments matter?

Did you know?

- The average male spends nearly all his health care dollars in the last year of his life trying to stay alive.

Do you grasp what is happening to your life and your health?

- Are you ready to accept the consequences for your decisions (or lack thereof)?
- When you die, get sick, or lose your zest for life (energy), your family and loved ones will have to pick up the slack. Are they ready to accept the consequences?
- When an illness comes knocking on your door and your world nearly shatters, will you be ready to hold it together with the strong foundational knowledge you gained?

Based upon what you know today, what changes do you need to make?

- Are you set up for success or failure to live a full life?
- Do you believe that you can do anything with God on your side? If not, I leave you with His word:
  - *"And my God will meet all your needs according to the riches of his glory in Christ Jesus."* Philippians 4:19 (NIV)
  - *"I can do all this through him who gives me strength."* Philippians 4:13 (NIV)

Are you ready?

- Are you motivated to live longer, healthier, and happier? If so, how motivated are you?
- What will make you successful in achieving better outcomes?
- Who can you depend on to support your goals and be your accountability partner?
- When can you start making changes in your life?
- Are you worth it?
- Are your loved ones worth the effort to create change in your life to enhance theirs?
- What stands in your way of achieving your goals? What can you do about it? Who can help?

Now, what are you going to commit to today?

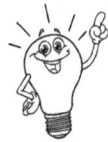

Do You Know?

Long Life with Low Insulin

What do all the longest living organisms have in common? Low insulin levels! Put simply, the less carbohydrates consumed, the less insulin secreted, the healthier you will be and the longer you are likely to live.

CHAPTER 7

WHAT ARE SOME EXTRAS I CAN DO?

"All truth passes through three states. First,
it is ridiculed. Second, it is violently opposed.
Third, it is accepted as self-evident."
Arthur Schopenhauer

CONGRATULATIONS!

YOU NOW HAVE SOME OF the information you need to live a very long and full life on your terms! Your story of life has already changed thanks to the knowledge you received in this book. You are now ready to take this information and put it into action in your life. As promised, I gave you information and shared ideas on a framework for a better future.

It is my hope that you learned not only more about the body and how it works, but more about yourself and what is happening to you. It is time to get serious about your health before it becomes compromised or before you start aging meaninglessly. There are root causes to what you are feeling, and you can do something about it! There are answers!

God created a masterpiece when you were born. Your body can do so much more than you can ever imagine or will challenge it to do. So, begin your journey to radiant health by tapping into the healing power within you. There are so many stories of miraculous healing, but you likely won't become one of them unless you set yourself on a path to healing through the power of knowledge.

I challenge you to develop your own protocol for living a radiant life full of good health, vitality, and longevity. Yes, you have the power within you, and now you have been equipped with the knowledge throughout this book. Don't stop here, though—tap into other resources to learn more about your health. You can visit my website at www.DrJoeyJones.com for more information, which I post regularly. Aside from that, grab more books and keep your learning alive! See my recommended reading section in the pages to follow!

Before You Go

As mentioned earlier in the book, it is critical to have a vision for ourselves—a vision of good health, vitality, and longevity. This vision can guide you to understand what you desire to achieve in order to realize the vision.

What does radiant health look like to you?

Seriously, close your eyes and ask yourself what radiant health looks like to you. Grab that vision of yourself and fix it in your mind.

- What do you see yourself doing?
- What are you wearing?
- Who is around you?
- What do you look like in the picture of radiant health?
- Where are you in the picture?
- What is different about you?
- How do you feel in the picture?
- What do you recognize in the picture from where you are today or your past?
- What is new in the picture?

Getting clear in your mind about the vision you have for yourself is a key first step to achieving that vision. You have taken that critical first step. If you can see this picture in your mind clearly, keep it in focus throughout your day. This picture is your "why" as to the hard work ahead of you on the journey towards vitality and longevity.

Now that you have put in the hard work to figure out what you are trying to achieve, let's put some words down on paper to clarify your vision. Describe what you are trying to achieve according to that picture. A few examples you can draw from are below:

- I am a strong and healthy individual full of energy. My hair is healthy and full of bounce, my skin is flawless, my body has definition, my smile is bright, and my inside health is just as good as my outside.
- I am healthy and strong—confident, resilient, and full of energy.
- I can play with my children or grandchildren for hours without becoming tired.
- I am working out with cardio and weights at a gym four times a week and the results are really starting to show—more muscle, less fat, more energy, more mental clarity, and a happier mood.
- I am staying active and able to live independently long into what others consider "old age."
- I am a go-getter in life, excited about what the day will bring. I no longer wish to stay in bed.
- I am leaping out of bed in toe-stubbing excitement each day to experience life's wonders.

Once you have your vision statement, consider writing it down on sticky notes and posting those everywhere you look: the bathroom mirror, refrigerator, computer, car, calendar, or on top of your keys that you grab every day! Having this reminder is important to do the hard work, day in and day out, choice by choice, to have a better life full of radiance!

There is More!

Now that you are clear on where you are going, you must figure out what it is that will get you there. Pull out a piece of paper or journal to start diving into what you need to do to take your life in the direction of radiance. Now, again, write your vision out on the top of the page. This is what is your driving force to get you to where you are going.

Now, ask yourself, how can you get there? Based upon the materials in this book, what are the key steps you need to take to get you closer to your vision of radiance? To figure this out, we should first define what is getting in your way.

Write down the question, "What is getting in the way of my vision for a radiant life?" Take five to 10 minutes to list everything that you can think of right now. You can revisit this question regularly, as the answers will change over time as you make changes in your life.

Share your questions during one of my webinars or Zoom classes. Schedules located on www.DrJoeyJones.com.

Examples to get you thinking:

- I have not carved out time in my schedule for things like walking, going to the gym, or stretching.
  - Tip: You likely won't be consistent with any key changes unless you get control over your time.

- I don't have any time to do anything for myself.
  - Tip: Create a short duration, high-energy, high-intensity program—start with 20-minute intervals.

- I am too tired to do anything!
  - Tip: Yes, today you are tired. However, if you start making changes today, you will be less tired in your future. The sky is the limit on what you can do as you find more energy.

- I start plans off strong, but then I get distracted.
  - Tip: This is why a plan and schedule are so critical.

- I am not healthy enough.
    - Tip: You will never be healthier unless you make changes. You will only continue to deteriorate under an unhealthy lifestyle and mindset. Make changes, even if they are small. There is always something you can do to better your health. Start there. Like climbing that mountain, the vision of your accomplishment is waiting over the next crest. Be patient. Be consistent.

The Challenge

OK, now that you know what is standing in your way, it is time to take steps to ensure they don't continue to stand in your way. It is time to plan and then act on your plan! By reading this material and other valuable material, you know many things that you can do to improve your health and overall well-being. It is now time to put this information to work for you!

What are you willing to do to get from where you are today to where you want to be?

Let's begin a 21-Day Challenge to reset your life and get you on the right track to better health and longevity.

21-Day Challenge Steps:

1. Develop your own 21-Day Challenge:
    a. Write a list of goals to take you closer to your vision. Examples include:
        i. Have a regular fitness program that incorporates yoga, walking, and weight training.
        ii. Walk five miles (at one time) at least three days per week. Maybe start with one mile ... it's OK, the key is to start.
        iii. Stay well-hydrated.

b. Determine what actions can support your goals.

    i. Set up a plan of five things you want to do daily (or stop doing) to get on a better path to a radiant life. Examples include:

1. Drink approximately 80 (plus) ounces of water each day.
2. Go to bed no later than 10 p.m. (start your bedtime routine at 9:30 p.m.).
   a. If you don't have a bedtime routine, I highly recommend one.
3. Shower every day upon rising to get your body going.
4. Spend at least 30 minutes a day reading a book.
5. Wake up at the same time every day (early enough to get a little "me time").
6. Take your supplements as directed (multiple times a day).
7. Eat at least two different colored vegetables each day.
8. Replace one hour of TV time a day with your passion, whether it is stretching, reading, journaling, dancing, or listening to music.
9. Don't weigh daily. Get healthy, then weigh. Consider weighing once per week.
10. Reduce by one soft drink (or cold beverage) per day, if that applies.
11. Reduce snacking.

c. Create a list of other actions you want to incorporate into your week that will further your ability to achieve your goals. Examples include:

    i. Weight training three to four times a week—short durations.

    ii. Walking on the beach two times a week (lucky you).

    iii. Going to yoga two times a week (if you are fit enough).

d. Now that you have this list, write up a schedule on how you can incorporate these activities and put them on your calendar.

e. If you find an accountability partner, give them your daily list of activities and your schedule. Set up regular touchpoints with them to go over your progress, discuss your challenges, ask for advice, or get encouragement.

   i. For instance, you could have a quick five-minute call daily or 15 minutes to check in two to three times a week.

2. Now that you know what to do, commit to your 21-Day Challenge:
   a. Calendar your kickoff date.
   b. Share it with friends.

Don't overwhelm yourself with committing for a lifetime. Commit for 21 days and see how it goes. Write about your journey in a journal to see how you transform (in both mental and physical ways). At the end of the 21 days, evaluate how you did, what stood in your way, and what you learned. Celebrate your successes. Then determine if the vision still holds true and if you need to make any adjustments. Then, press repeat! Take a moment and acknowledge your accomplishments. Enjoy the view for a moment!

If you need any support in developing your 21-Day Challenge, I am here to help you be successful. You don't have to do it alone if you are not comfortable. I have many resources on my website, but I also engage individually with people wanting more for their life. It may be that you need support in developing a plan or you just need some hired accountability to have some skin in the game. Whatever it is that you need, I am here for you. You CAN do this!

You don't have to make "lifetime" changes; just make small changes for a lifetime! Take life in bite-sized increments rather than solving everything all at once. I think this approach will make your more successful than doing a complete overhaul, which can often overwhelm us!

Your Reflection Corner

Chapter 7: What Are Some Extras I Can Do?

What would you do for a better tomorrow? When you look around, you may see young people suffering from things previously expected during old age. I do. I also see young people giving into bad health as if it is just another day. You have also likely seen how people in their 40s are living like they are in the 60s, and those in their 60s are living like they are in their 80s—slowing down, getting old before their time, not pushing themselves, or giving up.

I want more for you than disease, premature aging, and giving up on your health objectives. Don't you?

... Do you want to add years to your life expectancy?

... Do you want to improve how you feel during your golden years and before?

... Do you want to increase the things you can do now or in later years compared to others?

... Do you want to live as long as you can for your loved ones?

... Do you want to delay or avoid being dependent on your children?

... Do you want to continue to experience the spice of life throughout the remainder of your years?

Commit to the 21-Day Challenge and see everything in your life start to change. I like 21 days because it is not too short or too long. It's just the right amount of time.

I am excited about your journey to a better tomorrow. You've got this! Start today! An easy way to start right away is my 21-Day

Cleanse and Detox Toward Radiant Health. In three short weeks, you will have already significantly begun your transformation toward a new you.

Do You Know?

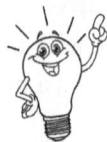

Youthful Complexion

Thymus gland supplementation can help.

Youthful skin, the so-called thymic complexion, is witnessed to the effect of the thymus gland promoting the youthful epidermis of children (i.e., "smooth as a baby's butt"). It accomplishes this phenomenon by its association with phospholiping, which together remove protein waste byproducts from connective tissue.

The key to preventing sun damage is to avoid calcium tissue loss caused by the sun's rays. Excess exposure to sunlight draws calcium from the tissue (skin) and transfers it into the blood, which results in no shielding protection due to calcium loss in the skin. Calcium works in our skin much like an eggshell. It acts like a layer of armor, which protects what is inside or underneath us. This is where the magic of vitamin F, better known as polyunsaturated fatty acids, comes to the rescue.

Examples are fish oils and flaxseed. These fats help to drive calcium from the blood and back into skin tissue for protection from UV light damage. And it does this without all the chemical toxicity and rancid oil absorption of sunscreens. These polyunsaturated fatty acids also help to reverse sunburn damage to tissues. This same physiological reaction of leaching calcium out of our tissue is why fever blisters are so common after overexposure to the sun, such as on beach trips or skiing vacations.

When tissue calcium is not in adequate supply in the skin, viruses are much more capable of expressing themselves, resulting in embarrassing canker sores. To prevent this, try using an ionized calcium supplement like calcium lactate, because cheap calcium supplements like calcium carbonates will not work. Add a supplement of fish oil or flaxseed oil before sun exposure.

Again, these oils help drive the calcium into the tissue for maximum absorption. The anti-aging benefits of these polyunsaturated fatty acids are well documented as is their ability to preserve chromosome telomere longevity by up to 33%. This results in improved cellular life span and improved longevity of all cells, including skin and hair care!

CHAPTER 8

CONCLUSION

I WROTE THIS BOOK FROM A place of "Healer, first heal thyself." This was the title of a paper I had first written shortly after graduating from Chiropractic College. I understood I had some healing of my own to do first. I was physically fit by most standards (such as blood pressure, body fat, blood work profiles, and physical appearances), but was I truly healthy? I wasn't feeling it so much anymore. I knew a change had to come. I knew I had to walk the walk and refill those dopamine receptor sites with something positive once again. So, I sat down quietly, one on one with my spirit, and signed my own accountability act. I knew these were things I needed to change for the ones I loved, but first I would have to change for my friend in the mirror: myself.

I had always been a social drinker—and yes, I drank heavily. Then 2020 and COVID hit. Like so many others, I found myself still drinking, but without the social setting. This was perhaps due to the lockdown. However, no excuses will be made by me. So, with encouragement from those in my inner circle, I entered into a detox program.

Personally, I am NOT a procrastinator. This meant trying to *ease off* my consumption approach did not work for me. If I was going to quit something, then I had to quit. Three days after entering detox, and three valium per day to ease my detox, I was released!

Welcome to the real world. How did I respond?

After my release came a test for my inner self. It was high time to go within, or I was surely destined to go without. There within me was my higher power, Jesus Christ, just as He had promised He would be. It was now and with the power He invested in me that I saw it was "time to turn back the hands of time." Time to slow down my biological merry-go-round and tame my telomeres before my health train ran off its tracks. Time to get this book out before I suffocate in silence of the lessons learned. I hope you will find something in this book you can use in your journey toward radiant health.

I'm both blessed and honored to be in a position to help others become empowered in their quest for better health. I help those willing to step out of the box of disease care and honor their right to control the future in optimal physical and mental possibilities relating to their health. No longer fearing uncertainty, loss of control, apprehension, or disbelief in their ability to make informed decisive decisions concerning their overall health for the years ahead.

Choices

Every day begins with a choice. Every one of us makes hundreds of choices each day. The dawn of each new day brings upon us a choice, an opportunity to jump out of bed with enthusiasm or to slumber for a little while longer. It is ours to choose. Either way, you have made a choice. Every situation we face in life, we will decide to either be proactive or reactive to that moment and situation in time. Proactive means we exercise our ability to choose our own response. The one area you have total responsibility and control over is in the ability to be proactive. Otherwise, we leave ourselves vulnerable to the alternative reaction of being reactive to our failure. That is a powerful ability.

As much as we may like to blame someone or something else (whether it be our genetics, our insurance company, our primary care provider, family, or friends), how we respond is totally on us. We can either be proactive (control) or reactive (controlled). How we prepare ourselves for the circumstances that lie ahead is under our control as well. Proactive if we choose, or we can leave circumstance to chance and respond reactively. I'll take my odds on the former any day.

I choose to be proactive because it is my choice. It's a power and freedom that belongs to me. Proactive, or reactive—we choose to be either one or the other. Proactive or reactive. Nobody else gets to choose your response. Not your doctor, not your insurance carrier, not your significant other, not the pharmaceutical companies. How powerful is that?

Every day, we all receive chances for new opportunities for choice. Choices that will empower you with knowledge. It was your choice to pick up this book and read it. Knowledge brings power, and power brings control—control to choose proactive responses to your health choices.

Choose your own thoughts and make your own decisions. You are the captain of your physical and emotional well-being, and the master of your fate. Remember, you have the capacity to choose. Choose a healthy life! Choose happiness! Choose love!

Purpose

Sometimes we just need a purpose. Kendall Layman, author of *The Gooder Life in Layman's Terms*, states: "Purpose keeps our paths from veering off into many directions." If you need a purpose for making a change in life and becoming healthier, how about that reflection staring back at you in the mirror? Take some time each day and take care of your best friend in the mirror. That reflection has been with you since the beginning, through thick and thin. It deserves your best. When you take it for a meal, take it to the best. You deserve it.

If you take care of that reflection, it is guaranteed that it is going to take care of you. So, in your search for a purpose in life, how about focusing on that best friend looking back at you every day? The one that is always there for you, out in front, guiding you through while also always having your back.

Have you got a little time for it today? Maybe 30 minutes to play at the gym. Take a walk with your spouse or child. Have a little one-on-one time. Maybe dance like no one's watching. Enjoy a few good meals each day. It's said that we value the things we do in life, not the things *we say* we value. Do you value your reflection as much as it does you? Congratulations if you are one of the those who's answer is, "Oh hell (heck) yes!"

Reaching Your Goal for Radiant Health

Reaching your goals toward radiant health can sometimes be compared to climbing a mountain. Accomplishments tend to occur step by step. You do not really experience much progress as it's happening. You are engulfed in the process of creating it, and much of the ground covered and the accomplishments you gain along the way are fairly invisible to you until you reach an overlook or a higher level of health along the way.

But once you stand up and look out over your accomplishments, your success rings out to everyone within earshot, with endless detailed stories about your accomplishments, how you achieved them, and how you ultimately reached your summit of radiant health!

Your Reflection Corner

Chapter 8: Conclusion

Have you committed to taking steps towards better health, vitality, and longevity?

If you are still contemplating what changes to make, consider these questions:

- How would you describe your current season of life?
- What is one thing you can complete in the morning every day to improve your overall wellness?
- What can you intentionally commit to and complete on a daily basis?
- What one habit can you simplify to be more consistent?
- What type of person do you want to become? What changes do you need to make to become that person and achieve that goal?
- Who are you ready to become? What can you do today to help you get there?

RECOMMENDED
READING BY DR. J

***Again, do not believe everything you read, or hear. Verify the
information yourself here!***

*The Magic of Cholesterol Numbers: A step away from the cholesterol-
lowering drugs* by Sergey A. Dzugan, MD, PhD, and Konstantine S.
Dzugan

*Malignant Medical Myths: Why Medical Treatment Causes 200,000
Deaths in the USA Each Year* by Joel M. Kauffman, Ph.D.

Any book written by David Perlmutter M.D.

*Wheat Belly: Lose the Wheat, Lose the Weight, and Find Your Path
Back to Health* by William Davis, M.D.

*Protein Power: The High-Protein/Low Carbohydrate Way to Lose
Weight, Feel Fit, and Boost Your Health-in Just Weeks!* By Michael R.
Eades, M.D. & Mary Dan Eades, M.D.

*Primal Body, Primal Mind: Beyond Paleo for Total Health and a Longer
Life* by Nora T. Gedgaudas and Nora Gedgaudas

Any book written by Dr. Royal Lee DDS

Any book written by Gabor Mate, M.D.

Testosterone for Life: Recharge Your Vitality, Sex Drive, Muscle Mass, and Overall Health by Abraham Morgentaler, M.D.

Maximize Your Vitality & Potency for Men Over 40 by Lenard Lane M.D. and Jonathan V. Wright Ph.D.

Lessons Learned... Through No Words at All by Kimberly Kelsoe Hawkins

Iodine: Why We Need It, Why You Can't Live Without It by David Brownstein

The Slow Burn Fitness Revolution: The Slow Motion Exercise That Will Change Your Body in 30 Minutes a Week by Fredrick Hahn M.D., Michael R. Eades M.D., & Mary Dan Eades M.D.

The Inflammation-Free Diet Plan: The scientific way to lose weight, banish pain, and prevent disease, and slow aging By Monica Reinagel

The Telomere Effect: A Revolutionary Approach to Living Younger, Healthier, Longer by Elizabeth Blackburn Ph.D., & Elissa Epel Ph.D.

Nutrition and Physical Degeneration by Weston A. Price DDS.

Good Calories, Bad Calories: Fats, Carbs, and the Controversial Science of Diet and Health by Gary Taubes

Why We Get Fat: And What to Do About It by Gary Tabues

A New Breed of Doctor by Alan H. Nittler M.D.

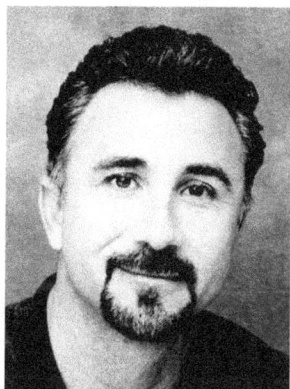

Dr. Joseph Jones is a Board-Certified Chiropractic Physician with more than 32 years of experience helping patients treat, prevent, and reverse musculoskeletal and degenerative diseases. He utilizes safe, non-toxic, non-invasive treatments that enhance the body's ability to heal itself and concentrates on a physiological approach to health and healing. These therapies are proving to be the present treatments of choice, as evidenced by society's monumental shift towards complementary alternative medicine. Dr. Jones helps patients foster these connections through his program of balancing body chemistry, nutrition, and lifestyle choices.

Dr. Jones educates readers about the shortcomings of conventional medicine and provides practical guidance for achieving vibrant health. He offers a comprehensive range of strategies, including nutrition, exercise, stress management, and the incorporation of holistic therapies to help readers take control of their well-being. These actionable steps empower individuals to make informed decisions and prioritize their health amidst an increasingly profit-driven healthcare system.

One of the book's strengths lies in Dr. Jones's ability to communicate complex medical concepts in a manner that is accessible to both healthcare professionals and readers. He skillfully breaks down intricate topics, making them easily understandable and relatable to everyday life.